body
wise

body
wise

10 steps to permanent
weight loss and well-being

Dr John Briffa

Daily Mail columnist

CICO BOOKS

London

Dedication

For my patients, who have taught me so much over the
years and were the inspiration behind this book.

Acknowledgements

This book would not have been possible without the help of some very special people. I would especially like to thank:

My wonderful parents, for supporting me ceaselessly in whatever I do. Thanks for being there and giving without question.

Hazel Courteney, for being such a wonderful, selfless friend and for inspiring so much of my work.

Debbie Sapstead, my fantastic assistant, for her tireless organization and sense of humour. Thanks for keeping me going over the last few months of writing this book.

Cindy Richards at Cima Books, for a great editing job and for accommodating my increasingly demanding and pedantic requests.

Dr John Stirling, for teaching me and continuing to teach me such an enormous amount about nutritional medicine.

Chris Williams, for being a great mate and for inspiring much of the chapter on exercise.

Jean Gollner, for reading through the manuscript and keeping my enthusiasm up with your encouragement.

And last, but not least, to Nellie, for giving me the room to do what I want to do, and for keeping me going with a never-ending stream of bright ideas.

Contents

Why BodyWise?

I know what you're thinking; do we really need another diet book? After all, go to the health section of any bookshop and you will find shelves heaving under the weight of books which claim to offer the solution to our ever-growing problem with excess weight and obesity. From high fibre to low fat, food combining to fasting, the sheer number and variety of weight loss regimes out there is simply mind-boggling. Actually, despite the glut of weight-loss books which do exist, the evidence that they are doing anyone any good is singularly thin on the ground. Statistics clearly show that the vast majority of people who lose weight on a diet put it all back on in time, and the percentage of overweight and obese individuals in many developed countries is set to double every seven years. Clearly, we are losing our battle with the bulge.

For me, excess weight is not a condition in itself, but a symptom of some underlying imbalance. What is more, the precise nature of this imbalance varies from individual to individual. Just as a car may stop running due to many reasons such as lack of fuel, faulty spark plugs or a problem with the transmission, many potential factors may underlie an individual's problem with weight. For one person, excess weight may be related to undesirable reactions to food and an undiagnosed thyroid problem. For another, it may be rooted in toxicity within the body and a problem with inefficient breathing. The secret to getting to grips with a weight problem is first to understand what's causing it, and then to correct it. That's what *BodyWise* is all about.

In this book I have set out the 10 core factors which are most likely to underlie a person's weight problem. Each chapter deals with a distinct approach to weight loss and well-being. The first chapter looks at the psychology surrounding weight and weight loss issues, and gives you tips on how to use your mind and attitude to catalyze change. The second chapter deals with the pitfalls of dieting, and why the secret to losing weight for many individuals is not to eat less, but to eat more. The remaining chapters deal with the other fundamental themes of food sensitivity, blood sugar balance, low thyroid function, toxicity in the body, fat intake, yeast overgrowth, inefficient breathing and exercise.

Now, not all of these factors are necessarily going to be relevant to you. The real purpose of this book is to allow you to identify those factors that *do* apply to you, and then give you the tools you need to correct them. You may come to find that your excess weight is caused by only one mechanism. Then again, perhaps several are playing a part in your personal weight problem. For many individuals, I find that three or four major factors are at work.

What this book essentially asks of you is to spend some time analyzing what is going on in your body and mind, and this task can be challenging. Weight-loss books which advocate a 'one size fits all' approach and tell you precisely what to eat, sometimes on a daily basis, are generally easy to follow and straightforward. However, if you are reading this book, there's a good chance you've tried one or more of these approaches in the past, and found that the results came up short. If this is the case, then you have yet to address the true underlying causes of your weight issue. Only by doing this can you expect to lose weight and enhance your health in a permanent, pervasive way.

BodyWise is really about taking control of your health. Too often, during my time as a doctor, I saw patients who were poorly informed about their condition, and had little or no say in their treatment regimes. Most patients simply had no idea of what was underlying their health issue. How then could they possibly be expected to take positive steps to help themselves? Seeing how passive and disempowered patients often were was a major trigger in my leaving conventional medicine.

Having originally planned a career in surgery, I suddenly found myself without a job or an income. To keep the wolf from the door, I spent some months doing locums as a junior doctor in hospital medicine. I travelled to a variety of hospitals in and around the south-east of England, filling in for doctors on leave, while I contemplated my next move. On one such posting, I was to meet a patient who changed my life forever.

I was working as a junior surgeon in Newmarket. On my second morning there, my job was to assess a number of patients who were due for minor operations that afternoon. One of the patients I saw that day was an elderly man who had come in for a hernia repair. Although he was in his seventies, he didn't look older than sixty. Individuals of his age normally have some significant past medical history such as high blood pressure or diabetes, but he had none. In fact, he had never been in hospital before. He was physically robust, and had a marvellous disposition too. This man enjoyed life, and talked at length about his love for his wife, which was as strong then as it was when they had first met some 50 years earlier.

I was so struck by this man's physical and emotional well being, that I asked him to what he attributed his youthfulness and vigour. He proceeded to tell me that he had always eaten a healthy diet, including organic vegetables which he grew on an allotment. Most days, he cycled several miles to and from this allotment, and worked hard tending it too. He also confessed to taking nutritional supplements, in particular the mineral selenium which is known to have anti-ageing and cancer-protective effects. He would often read and listen to the radio, and was still very interested in learning new things and developing his mind.

During my meeting with this man, it dawned on me that perhaps the real secret to health was not so much a matter of luck, but more to do with how we live our lives. I began to think that our experience of life might have a lot to do with the food we eat, the activity we take, and what goes on in our heads. This might not sound like much of a revelation, but at the time this was a new concept for me. My medical training taught me to view illness largely as an inevitable consequence of life, and something that could only really be combated using drugs or surgery. My chance meeting with this wonderful man had triggered me into a new way of thinking, and posed questions that needed answering.

I wanted to know why it was we became sick, and started to look for ways in which we could prevent and treat illness using natural methods and treatments. I began buying books about nutrition and natural health. I read voraciously. I would visit libraries and look-up research papers. Over the next few months, I read dozens of books and hundreds of research papers. The more I learnt, the more I realized there was to learn. A whole new way of practising medicine was opening up to me and I was like a kid in a sweet shop.

Very quickly, I made up my mind that my job would be to make this information available to the public in any way I could. The problem was, I had no concept of how to do this. My experiences at medical school had been so confined that I did not know that nutritional therapy nor nutritionists existed, and naively imagined that I was embarking on some sort of lone pilgrimage into the field of nutrition.

Knowing of my new-found interest, a good friend introduced me to a doctor who owned a chain of weight-loss clinics. As I was ignorant of what was going on in the area of nutrition and natural medicine, I assumed that these clinics were where doctors who were interested in nutrition ended up. I was keen to use my recently acquired knowledge to help individuals, and this seemed like an ideal opportunity.

So, a day or two a week, I began to consult clients, whose sole aim was to lose weight. Each individual was recommended the same diet, a high-protein, low-carbohydrate diet, backed up with appetite suppressants in most cases. This approach worked for the majority of people. Weight loss would usually come, occasionally in quite spectacular fashion. I was satisfied that what we offered at the clinic was a safe and effective approach to losing weight. Then the trouble started.

After some months of working this way, I became aware that many individuals who were previously losing weight, were now failing to do so. Often their weight would plateau at a level way above what they considered to be desirable. We had a strict rule at the clinic; no consistent weight loss, no appetite suppressants. So, many clients would inevitably fall off the horse, often to return some months later, usually heavier than before. It occurred to me that something wasn't right. Somehow, we were failing to address the true causes of these people's weight problems.

Around this time, I read a thick tome on the subject of obesity. One of the basic premises in the book was that our weight is largely genetically determined, and there's not that much we can do to change it. The book explored the concept that our weight is essentially dictated by our genes because of certain evolutionary factors. When we were hunter-gatherers thousands of years ago, food could often be in short supply, and some of us would perish due to starvation. However, individuals with the capacity to put on and retain fat were more likely to survive in times of famine, and therefore stood a better chance of reproducing. In this way, the book argued, many of us may have inherited genes which mean we are destined to become overweight. If this were true, then perhaps I was deluding myself in thinking that weight and other health issues were really more about nurture than nature.

I began thinking about the rapidly increasing rates of excess weight and obesity in the Western world. Could these depressing statistics really be the result of unfortunate genetic inheritance? Ask any genetic scientist and they'll tell you that genes change very, very slowly. It takes literally thousands of years for significant changes to occur in the genetic pool of the human species. If this is the case, then we simply can't explain our burgeoning weight problem with genetics. The problems that we are now seeing with excess weight which have arisen in the last few decades can only have come out of changes in dietary, activity-related and psychological factors. Yes, we may have inherited genes which may make us prone to weight gain, but the expression of these genes is *clearly* largely related to our lifestyle habits.

Having come full circle with my thinking, I set about attempting to find more precisely what was really at the root of my clients' weight issues. I was becoming acutely aware that while a certain diet might suit one individual, this was not necessarily the case for another. While many individuals lost weight on the high protein diet, others did not. Why not? Clearly, not all overweight individuals were overweight for the same reason, and it seemed likely that a range of different factors were at play. It was around this time that I became interested in many of the concepts which are explored in this book. I started to tailor my clients' dietary and lifestyle approaches according to their individual needs.

Low and behold, individuals who had battled with their weight for many years started to lose weight once again, but this time things were different. By understanding better the reasons why they were overweight, they seemed more able to make permanent changes in their lives. Maybe for the first time, many clients could see the point to taking a new course, and were consequently happy and enthusiastic about change. Best of all, taking an informed, individualized approach led so many of these individuals to permanent weight loss and true well-being.

In time, I identified the concepts and strategies which were of most use in helping my clients overcome their weight and health issues. My experience with thousands of clients has been condensed into this book. What took me literally years to discover, *BodyWise* gives you the opportunity to learn in just a few hours. Armed with the information it contains, you can wise up to what's happening in your body, and take the steps you need to conquer your weight and health issues – *for good.*

A word about supplements

In this book I have recommended vitamins, minerals, herbs and other natural agents that have been found to help correct body imbalances and improve well-being and vitality. Because I believe it is important for you to understand the specific effects of natural substances in the body, I have listed them individually and included some information about each (see page 183). However, we know from experience that natural agents work synergistically, and so have the most impact when taken together. Where relevant, therefore, I have recommended combination supplements that contain a blend of agents specifically formulated with a particular problem in mind. Taking nutrients as combination supplements is generally easier and cheaper than buying and using them individually.

I have always made it my policy not to derive financial benefit from the recommendation and sale of supplements. Even in my practice I do not sell supplements, but suggest my clients buy them from the manufacturer or a health food store. I have no commercial interest in the products contained in the book, but I have included them to help take the guesswork and error out of finding a nutritional supplement that is right for you.

And finally, please remember that supplements are a useful adjunct to, not a replacement for, a healthy diet and lifestyle. Bear in mind that any supplement will be most effective when used in conjunction with the other recommendations outlined in this book.

1

Think Slim

Weight loss is often viewed as a taboo subject. Many of us feel embarrassed to admit that we are not comfortable with our shape or size. Being overweight can cause many of us to feel as if we've failed somehow and that we're just not making the grade. The effect our weight can have on our feelings of confidence and self-worth is amazing. While there are many good medical reasons for losing weight – a reduced risk of heart disease, cancer, diabetes and arthritis to name a few – the main issue for most would-be slimmers is that they simply are not happy with how they look and feel.

While we doctors may warn of the hazards associated with being overweight, what is often ignored is the fact that this is essentially an emotive issue, bound up with attitudes that relate to our body image and self-esteem. There is no doubt that excess weight, and failed attempts at losing it, are big issues for a great number of people. Just look at the statistics:

● **A 1997 survey revealed that 47% of women and 29% of men of average weight for height and sex view themselves as overweight (1).**

● **The same survey found that 84% of women and 58% of men reported having dieted to lose weight.**

● **66% of women are unhappy with their weight. This percentage in 1972 was 48%, representing an almost 40% increase in just 27 years (2).**

● It has been estimated that 80% of 10-year-old American girls have been on a diet (2).

● Anorexia nervosa affects one in 100 middle class teenage girls and young women. This figure can rise dramatically to one in 20 for those in body-conscious professions such as modelling, ballet dancing and sport.

Time to change

If your primary motivation for reading this book is weight loss, then there's a pretty good chance that you've recently had one of those body image experiences that has jarred you into taking action. Perhaps you've tried on a skirt or a pair of trousers that you could get into a few months ago but now find uncomfortably tight. Maybe you look longingly at the clothes featured in glossy magazines but feel you're just not the right shape and size to carry them off. Perhaps you choose your wardrobe with the idea of camouflaging as much of your body as is feasibly possible. Maybe you just feel overweight and out of condition and that you've 'let yourself go'. It could be that you feel a sense of shame or failure when you look at yourself in the mirror. Or maybe you cannot bear to look in the mirror at all. Is the truth of the matter that you just feel unloved and unlovable because of how you think you look?

The one common factor that binds these experiences together is that they all involve an element of self-criticism. So many of us judge our bodies very harshly and beat ourselves up when we feel we've failed in the body stakes. Ironically, while it may seem on the surface that being dissatisfied with your weight or shape is a good starting point for change, it is this negative attitude about yourself that may actually be perpetuating the problem.

Think slim

There's an old adage: 'What you resist, persists.' The idea here is that if you tend to focus on something in your life that you don't actually want, the very act of focusing on it causes it to perpetuate. Bearing in mind that many overweight people are involved in a continual battle with their body weight, it's no surprise that weight issues continue to abound.

One important way of getting around this problem is to change your whole mental tack. Instead of concentrating on not being overweight, why not try putting your energy into being slim. Sound the same? It's not. Essentially, human motivation is stronger if we are moving *towards* something *positive*, rather than attempting to move *away* from something *negative*. Taking steps towards being slim is more compelling, and also much less, emotionally draining than attempting to escape the problem of being overweight.

So, instead of getting locked into focusing on those physical attributes that you are not happy with, keep in mind the size and shape of the body you really want to have. If it's a trimmer waist and firmer thighs that you want, then that's the image to keep in mind as you go through your process of change. If you're looking to be fitter and healthier, then hold that as your ultimate goal. Form a very clear picture in your mind of how you want to look. Once you have achieved this, it's time to move onto the next stage.

Feel slim

Now that you have a positive image of the person you want to be, get excited about it! How would you feel if you were slim and healthy now? Plug into your new vision of yourself with all your senses, just as if you were that person right here, right now. Imagine how this new you would think and feel. Once you can truly see and feel this transformed image of yourself, it's time to take action.

Be slim

The third step to achieving a new body is to do something about it. Behave in a way that is in accordance with the person you see and feel. As much as possible, act in a manner that you would expect this transformed image of yourself to behave. Eat the health-giving foods you see the new you eating. Make a regular date with your exercise bike or running shoes. Stand tall in front of the mirror and be proud of how you look. Do anything and everything that is representative of the person you truly want to be. Playing at being transformed can be an incredibly powerful tool in bringing your aspirations into reality.

Make peace with yourself

Paradoxical though it may sound, the real key to changing into the person you want to be is to actually accept yourself for what you already are. As we have just discussed, the motivation for change is often rooted in issues concerned with body image. For so many the image they have of their body is based on self-criticism. The emotional burden this creates does nothing to speed the process of change. Remember: *what you resist, persists*. The irony is, if you are committed to change, then it really will help you to accept yourself as you are. Whatever your shape, take some time each day to celebrate the fact that you are who you are.

Accepting yourself for who you are does not mean that you don't have to endeavour to improve yourself or strive to achieve new goals. What it does mean is that you may find that positive change comes much more naturally and effortlessly when you stop judging and finding fault with your body. The drive for self-improvement is completely healthy, provided it comes from a place of self-love rather than a feeling of inadequacy.

Trust yourself

Another important element in any process of change is trust. After all, it is lack of trust that lets fear in. And fear of being overweight, as we have said, is the very thing that is likely to perpetuate the problem. Don't even bother questioning or feeling anxious about whether you are going to be able to lose the weight you want. Trust that you will.

Make friends with food

Most of the messages we get from health professionals regarding diet are essentially negative. A great deal of dietary advice given by doctors and dieticians is concerned with telling us what not to do. For example, you would have had to have spent the last few years living on Mars not to have got the message that eating a high-fat diet is not good for your weight or your health. And how many times have you read or heard about the potential hazards of eating too much sugar? Similar messages are common for everything from fast food to alcohol, chocolate to cheese. With so many negative messages all around us, it is no surprise that many of us have built very strong mental barriers to food.

So, individuals often go into a phase of dieting, hell-bent on avoiding 'fattening' foods. The problem here is that the mind-set of such an approach is based on not doing something, i.e. not eating unhealthy food. Yet, as we've already mentioned, concentrating on doing something, rather than on not doing something, is a much more powerful motivator for action. Rather than focusing on reducing or eliminating unhealthy foods from your diet, concentrate instead on increasing the amount of healthy foods that you do eat. You might be surprised to find just how effective this simple adjustment of thought is for reducing your feelings of deprivation and in maintaining your motivation.

Remember, while food may appear to be your undoing, it is also very likely to play a major part in your salvation. One of the chief aims of this book is to give you the opportunity to discover which foods are best suited to you if you want to achieve weight loss and health. If you tend to see food as something bad, may I suggest that you are very likely to benefit from viewing it in a more positive light. By seeing food as an ally in your quest to lose weight and regain your health, it can take much of the struggle out of the process.

Never say never

While on a diet, have you ever reached the end of a delicious restaurant meal and wanted to kill for a crème brûlée? Full of fat and sugar, you know in your heart that this seductive little pudding is only going to undo days of dietary control and restraint. I beg to differ. Contradictory though it may seem, having the crème brûlée may be very effective in moving you towards your personal health goal. How? By stopping those feelings of denial and deprivation that can sap the resolve of the most hard-bitten slimmer.

Imagine that you want to eat the crème brûlée but decide to deny yourself the pleasure. Maybe other people around the table are having a dessert, but you choose to go without. In such a situation you can start to resent your new lifestyle habits for denying you some of the pleasures of eating. As resentment builds, resolve generally declines, increasing the risk that you may end up giving up the whole thing and going back to how you were. However, there is another way.

Let's try to see the crème brûlée in a wider context. Maybe you decide to view it alongside all the food you have consumed in the last week. Hey, it's been a pretty good week, with lots of healthy foods, regular meals and a couple of exercise sessions to boot. Remind yourself that it's what you eat most of the time, not occasionally as special treats, that counts. So, eat your crème brûlée, enjoy it – savour it, even. You haven't done something terrible and you are not going to be banished to slimming hell. In your mind, resolve to carry on as usual, safe in the knowledge that you can have the occasional treat *and* lose weight.

Hunger has no role in weight loss

For many, dieting can be an empty experience. Ever since the calorie approach to dieting began in the 1930s, the core principle of most weight loss regimes has been eating less. Meals of a size barely big enough to satisfy a sparrow, together with lectures on the sin of eating between meals, are common features in most slimming plans. In the next chapter we'll be discussing why reducing the amount of food we eat can slow the metabolism and jeopardize our chances of long-term weight loss. We'll also be discussing how eating between meals can actually speed up weight loss, rather than scupper it. Prepare to have a few pre-conceived ideas about losing weight challenged.

However, right now, it's time to discuss the concept of hunger. Although hunger is a common experience for many would-be slimmers, I firmly believe that it has no part to play in weight loss. I often think that some people don't believe they can lose weight *unless* they spend a significant proportion of the day hungry. My take is that hunger is *never* an essential ingredient in the weight-loss mix.

By understanding your body and feeding it with healthy food, it is possible to shed pounds without pain. Part of this understanding is about getting to grips with hunger. To my mind, there are five principal types of hunger. Let's go through the cause and cure for each:

1. Plain old physical hunger

You're busy, it's 2.30 in the afternoon and you've skipped lunch. Your stomach is empty and has started to rumble. Food, and it doesn't really matter what, has suddenly become a priority. You could go without for a bit longer, but you would much prefer not to.

This is physical hunger, and every person on the planet will be familiar with this sensation. Coping with this type of hunger is easy: just eat. We'll be discussing exactly what to eat throughout the rest of the book.

2. Sweet and starch cravings

It's 4.30 in the afternoon, and despite having a big lunch, you're hungry again. Not that any old food will do, mind. You'd murder for something sweet – only a chocolate bar or biscuit will do.

This type of hunger may well be familiar to you and it indicates low levels of sugar in the bloodstream – also known as hypoglycaemia. It's a plain and simple fact that when the level of sugar in the body drops, there's a tendency for the body to crave foods that replenish sugar quickly. These include sweet-tasting foods and refined starchy carbohydrates such as white bread and pasta. By eating regularly, basing the diet around foods that give a sustained release of sugar into the body throughout the day, and supplementing with some essential nutrients, it is almost always possible to stop this type of hunger in its tracks. Read chapter 3, *Balance Your Blood Sugar*, to find out more.

3. Very specific cravings

You love bread and pasta and can't bear to be without them. In fact, bread and pasta feature in just about every meal and you feel as though something's missing if you eat a meal that does not include one of them. Given the choice between bread and potatoes, you'd go for bread every time.

Sometimes craving a specific food type can indicate that your body has a problem with it. Here, the body can react to one or more foods that can lead to problems with excess weight and ill-health in the long term. Strange though it may seem, some people have an uncanny attraction to the very foods they are sensitive to. For example, a penchant for bread and pasta can indicate a sensitivity to wheat. Children often exhibit this phenomenon – kids who love cheese or are wedded to the milk bottle are normally sensitive to dairy products. Read chapter 6, *Eliminate Your Allergies*, for information on food sensitivity, how to find your problem foods and what to do about it.

4. Cravings for nutrients

You know that red meat isn't the healthiest food in the world and prefer to eat chicken or fish. Every so often, though, you get a real yearning for beef. Somehow, your rational mind seems to be over-ridden and you suddenly find yourself ordering the steak, rather than the sea bass.

At times we may crave foods because our body is looking for the specific nutrients those foods contain. Craving red meat can be a sign of iron deficiency, for example. This mechanism explains why dogs sometimes eat grass and children can develop a strange fascination with dirt as a food. Another example is pica, where pregnant women get an overwhelming desire to eat something strange, such as coal – coal craving is usually a sign of an iron and/or calcium deficiency. Ensuring that you eat a good balanced diet (more about this throughout the book) with the addition of a good quality daily multivitamin and mineral will usually put a stop to these deficiency-related cravings.

5. Comfort eating

For you, eating is related to your emotions. Should you become upset or stressed, it's food you turn to first. When you're in an emotional turmoil, a big bar of chocolate or half a loaf of bread can disappear in rapid time. You eat healthily a lot of the time, but your eating habits can spin out of control when the pressure is on.

Eating that is triggered by emotional stress or upset in this way may be related to several factors. I suspect the major two are connected with social conditioning and brain biochemistry.

Social conditioning

Food is often used to pacify or reward children. Almost every child will have experienced being offered a 'treat' of chocolate, cake, biscuits or juice when they are upset. Such scenarios can be repeated hundreds, if not thousands of times during a child's formative years. Often, the end result is a child who sees food as something that induces a feeling of comfort. You can just imagine the potential for this continuing into adulthood. How many of us turn to food when we feel stressed or distressed? Within this book there is a lot of information that will allow you to develop a whole new relationship, not just with your body, but with your mind, too. Take on board the advice here, and there's a good chance you'll change your relationship with food forever.

Brain biochemistry

The brain contains chemicals called neurotransmitters that allow cells to communicate with each other. One of these neurotransmitters is called serotonin, which generally induces happy, feel-good emotions. Serotonin is the active constituent in many anti-depressants, such as Prozac. This chemical is manufactured in the brain from a substance called tryptophan, which itself is an amino acid found in the diet. Foods rich in tryptophan include meat, tofu, almonds, peanuts, pumpkin seeds, sesame seeds and tahini (sesame seed paste). The more tryptophan we have in the brain, the happier we are likely to be. Tryptophan is absorbed into the brain more efficiently if there is plenty of carbohydrate present. This mechanism could possibly explain why certain individuals crave sweet or starchy foods ('comfort foods') when they become emotionally upset or stressed.

If you think this process may be a factor for you, then you may benefit from taking a supplement called 5-hydroxytryptophan (5-HTP). Before tryptophan is converted into serotonin it is first converted into 5-HTP. Theoretically, 5-HTP should reduce tendencies to binge on carbohydrate foods, and some individuals have found 5-HTP beneficial for this reason. The normal recommended dose is 50mg, two or three times a day. 5-HTP is available from health food stores.

What's my target weight?

Many people embarking on a weight loss regime will often set themselves a target weight. The question is: how do you know what your ideal weight really is? Excess weight can be calculated in a number of ways. Probably the two most commonly used methods are the 'body mass index' and the 'body fat percentage'. Each measurement looks at weight in a slightly different way.

Body Mass Index

The Body Mass Index (BMI) is popular amongst members of the medical profession as a way of ascertaining the degree of an individual's weight problem. You can calculate your BMI by dividing your weight in kilograms by the square of your height in metres.

$$\frac{\textbf{Weight (Kg)}}{\textbf{Height (m)}^2}$$

The higher your BMI, the heavier you are. The following is a guide to medically determined bands that relate BMI to the risk of ill-health:

BMI Men		BMI Women
Less than 20	**underweight**	Less than 19
20 – 25	**healthy**	19 – 24
26 – 30	**overweight**	25 – 29
31 – 40	**obese**	30 – 40
More than 41	**very obese**	More than 41

The graph *(opposite)* allows you to easily calculate the BMI band you fall in.

Each of the above bands has a different implication for health, with the 'healthy' range obviously being the place to be. If you are underweight or overweight this may have negative consequences for your health. The more overweight you are, the worse the outlook is. However, one major failing of the BMI system of weight assessment is that it looks at overall body weight in relation to height, and is therefore not a very good guide to body make-up. People who are heavily muscled may have a high BMI, but that doesn't mean they are fat. It's not being over*weight* that is the problem, it's being over*fat*. Ascertaining your BMI does not necessarily allow you to distinguish between a problem with excess fat and a big build.

Another problem with the BMI system is that the healthy band is much too wide to be able to give the individual an idea of their ideal weight. For example, a 165cm (5'6") woman could be as light as 52 kg (8 st 2 lb) and as heavy as 65 kg (10 st 4 lb) and yet still be in the healthy band. The BMI is probably a useful guide to the likely health implications of your weight, but it has limitations as a tool for ascertaining your ideal weight.

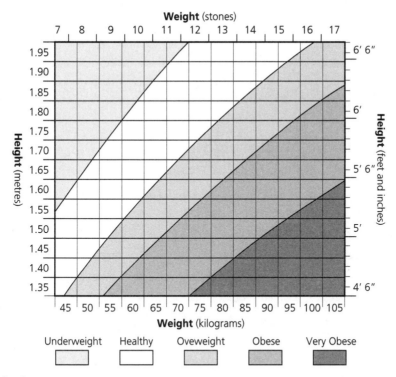

| | Underweight | Healthy | Oveweight | Obese | Very Obese |

Body fat percentage

By assessing the percentage of the body made up of fat, it is possible to distinguish between excess fat and a big build. The parts of the body other than fat (principally muscle, bone and water) make up what is termed the 'lean body compartment'. This tends not to change very much and in healthy individuals makes up between 80 and 85% of body mass. The body's fatty component, sometimes described as 'fat mass', is the bit we're essentially interested in. Our chief aim is to reduce the fat mass, while at the same time preserving our muscle bulk and bone strength.

BFPs (body fat percentages) are normally calculated from skin-fold thickness measurements taken with callipers at various sites over the body. Your BFP is often calculated as part of a health screen or gymnasium induction. Recently, weighing scales have become available which are designed to assess BFP by measuring the body's electrical resistance.

Ideal fat mass values for men and women are as follows:

Men: between 15% and 20% of total body mass

Women: between 17% and 23% of total body mass

While BFPs are great for assessing body make-up, for most of us they are mainly of theoretical interest. The fact is, very few of us are going to have an accurate assessment of our BFP, making setting an ideal weight through this form of assessment very unlikely.

So, what is my ideal weight?

It is my honest belief that the vast majority of individuals instinctively know what is a good weight for them, and that this is a relatively personal and individual issue. When a client asks me 'What weight should I be?' I say, 'What weight do you feel comfortable at?' Mostly, I get an answer such as, 'Well, I felt great at 9 stones' or 'I'd really like to get down to about 12 or 12½ stones'. My response to this is usually, 'Fine, let's aim for that then'. I am generally averse to the concept of using some formula or sophisticated piece of equipment to arrive at an ideal body weight. There really is too much individual variability in body type for this to work for everyone. What I see very often is that a slavish adherence to such methods of assessment can cause individuals to attempt to force themselves down to a weight which is difficult to attain and near impossible to maintain.

For me, unless there is some major issue with distorted body image (as in anorexia nervosa), then an individual's sense of his or her ideal weight or size really is the most appropriate target to aim for. My advice is not to be too stuck on a particular weight. Let's say you weigh 68 kg (10 st 10 lb) and have a target of 59 kg (9 st 4 lb). Now let's imagine you lose weight slowly and steadily get down to 60 kg (9 st 6 lb). You may feel great at this weight, but because you have not reached your target weight there may be a tendency to feel as if you've failed. Feelings of success are much more likely if you set your target weight as a range, in this case maybe 57 – 61 kg (9 – 9½ stone).

Keeping track

Once you have set some sort of target weight, how are you going to go about assessing your progress? The obvious start is to weigh yourself. While regular weighing may be a simple way of keeping a tab on your weight loss, I would keep the frequency of your weighing sessions to a minimum. The body can be prone to quite significant fluctuations in weight that may not have much to do with what you've eaten, and this can be misleading. For example, on a hot, dry day we can quite easily drop one or two kilograms (three or four pounds) because of dehydration. Conversely, during a low pressure spell the body will tend to retain water, causing our weight to rise. Daily weigh-ins may be too affected by such fluctuations to give an accurate guide to how you are doing. If you are going to use scales, I would like to suggest the following:

1. If you haven't already, get yourself a decent set of scales. The cheap, spring-loaded type is usually not sufficient for accurate measurement. Heavy duty (but rather expensive) spring based scales are much better. Another alternative is electronic scales. These are relatively inexpensive and generally do a good job. Put them on a hard, level surface for maximum accuracy.

2. Weigh yourself no more than once a week. Bearing in mind how misleading day-to-day fluctuations can be, weighing yourself more frequently than this does not make sense. I suggest you weigh yourself on the same day of the week, at about the same time, in the same state of dress (or undress).

3. Don't get too fixed on weight as the most important thing. I'm not sure why this is, but many individuals will often change shape and lose inches, only to find that the scales show only minimal weight loss. Remember here that the most important thing is that you feel and look better; what the scales say is really of only secondary importance, unless there is some pressing, medical need to lose weight.

Slow and steady, that's the way

All of us will be familiar with the claims of dietary regimes that paint pictures of pounds dropping off and fat melting away. It is not uncommon for individuals to lose several pounds in the first week of a very low calorie diet. Yet, the body will generally lose only half or a kilogram (one or two pounds) of weight per week in the form of fat, the rest is likely to be due to a loss of fluid and a reduction in glycogen stores (glycogen is the main form in which carbohydrate is stored in the body).

The real point of any weight loss programme is to lose fat. Even if you are eating a diet that is both individualized and healthy, don't be surprised if your weight loss is less than dramatic. Correct me if I'm wrong, but you didn't amass all your weight over a few weeks. Expecting it all to come off quickly may therefore be a tad unrealistic. Take comfort in the fact that individuals who lose weight slowly and steadily appear to do a much better job of maintaining their new weight when compared to crash dieters.

My body image lesson

In March of 1999 I spent a week on Captiva Island, Florida. I was part of a small team of British health professionals who had flown out to the States to teach a course on lifestyle management to employees of the consultancy firm PricewaterhouseCoopers. One of the other team members was Chris Williams, the trainer and exercise physiologist whose expertise I leant on to write the final chapter of this book. Chris and I go back a long way. In fact, we were at school together and have been friends for over 20 years. Chris is supremely fit and a former member of the British triathlon team. It won't surprise you to learn that Chris has quite a body. Lean and muscular, he really does embody the health and fitness message.

I have never been a great natural swimmer, so during our time in Florida I asked Chris to help me improve my swimming technique. In whatever spare time we had, Chris would patiently coach me in the outdoor pool, just a stone's throw from the conference centre. One day, after such a training session, Chris and I were sitting in our swimming shorts discussing some of the concepts for this very book. Being around Chris, it's easy to become self-conscious about your body. As we talked, I became increasingly aware of my own physical shortcomings. The fact is, Chris is taller than me, carries very little body fat and has an infinitely better physique. I could feel my sense of self-esteem start to ebb away. Then I started to think that however hard I tried, I was unlikely to ever swim as well as Chris. I was having a real confidence crisis, and the irony was that we were discussing the concept of self-acceptance at the time! Then I realized how crazy this was. I pulled myself up and started to focus on some more positive thoughts. So, I may not be an international athlete, but I'm fit and healthy and have been lucky enough to participate in many different sports and activities. Hey, and on top of all this, thanks to Chris, my swimming was improving every day! Almost instantaneously, the negative thoughts and self-doubt evaporated and I felt a renewed sense of contentment and optimism. This little episode was a clear reminder to me of just how important it is to retain a positive image of oneself through any process of learning and change.

Summary

- The primary issue of individuals wishing to lose weight is usually one of poor body image and low self-esteem.

- Concentrate as much as possible on an image of the person you want to be.

- Have a clear picture in your mind of the new you. Feel what it would be like to be that person – and then act it out.

- Stop judging and start accepting yourself.

- Trust that change will come.

- See food as an ally in your efforts to lose weight and improve your health.

- Be open to eating all foods, albeit in moderation. The key to health is balance and this rarely requires complete exclusion of anything.

- Resolve that you really don't have to be hungry to lose weight. Spend some time getting in touch with your hunger so that you can take the most appropriate steps to combat it.

- Set a realistic target weight, based on what you feel comfortable at.

- Aim for steady weight loss – and enjoy the process of change.

2

Eat More

If you've been in the dieting game a while, and even if you haven't, you'll probably think that eating less is a fundamental part of losing weight. But the fact is that while eating less usually does help to shift weight initially, the effects of food restriction may have undesirable consequences for weight loss in the long term. As you'll discover in this chapter, it is the very act of eating that assists the body to shed its unwanted fat stores. The key to losing weight for many people to is not to eat *less*, but *more*.

The widespread belief that a reduction in food consumption is a prerequisite for weight loss is based on the calorie principle of dieting. This principle was first put forward in 1930 by two doctors, Newburgh and Johnston, at the University of Michigan, USA. Their theory was that if we consume fewer calories than our body burns, then we are bound to lose weight. For instance, if our body burns, say, 2,500 calories in a day but we consume only 1,500, then a 1,000-calorie deficit results. To compensate, the body burns stored fuel to make up for this energy shortfall, and weight is therefore lost. Since the 1930s the medical profession has adhered to the idea that calorie reduction is the only effective way to lose weight.

Although apparently sound in theory, the calorie principle is dangerously simplistic. While calorie restriction will almost certainly produce some weight loss initially, this loss can be virtually unsustainable due to a variety of physiological and biochemical factors. Despite the medical profession's attachment to calorie-based dieting, no studies exist to suggest that it is effective for long-term weight loss at all. To understand why this is, it is important first to understand the relationship between food and the metabolism.

The fire within

The speed at which the body burns fuel is referred to as the 'metabolism'. To a large degree, the metabolic rate is governed by the function of the thyroid gland in the neck. To learn more about the importance of this gland in weight control and health, refer to chapter 4, *Keep Up the Heat*. Apart from the thyroid, the metabolism is also affected by other factors such as exercise and food. To understand how food affects our metabolism it is useful to think of the body as a sophisticated furnace, where the fire in the furnace represents the body's metabolism and the fuel for the fire represents food.

Imagine we've lit a fire that had been burning well but now seems to be dwindling somewhat. If we want to keep the fire going, we know we're going to have to put more fuel on it. A few coals or a couple of dry logs and soon the fire is burning well again. A similar effect happens in the body. When we eat, the fire within us – the 'metabolism' – increases, enhancing our fuel-burning potential.

Anyone cutting back on the amount of food they eat is likely to lose weight initially. After all, if we leave a fire without adding more fuel to it, the existing fuel gets burnt. However, eventually the flames go out and all we're left with is a few dying embers. The fuel-burning capacity of the fire is now greatly reduced. It's just the same in the body. When calories are restricted, the body soon becomes wise to the fact that food is in short supply and so it does its best to conserve any existing stores of energy. In effect, the body adjusts itself to the reduced supply and adapts by burning progressively less fat.

Some dieters think that skipping meals and going hungry must be the best way to lose weight. If we think for a moment about the fire inside us, then we can see just how mistaken this belief is. If we light a fire at breakfast time and don't fuel it in the middle of the day, what happens by the time we come back to the fire in the evening? The flame will be so low that the fuel we put on it in the evening will not burn easily at all. Skipped meals mean that our body is more likely to store subsequent meals as fat.

The real problems start once we start to increase our fuel intake again. Put more fuel on a fire that is almost out and it's likely that it will not burn at all well. There's a good chance that some of the fuel will end up unburnt. In the body, unburnt fuel tends to stick around as fat.

Now, if you're thinking that this theory is just that, there is scientific evidence to support it. In one study, rats were studied as they gained and lost weight. Each time these rats lost and regained weight, their metabolism progressively slowed. The weight loss in the second cycle was half as fast as it was in the first, and the weight came back three times as quickly (1). This effect has also been confirmed in humans (2).

The bottom line for long-term weight loss is that it's not how much you eat, but what you eat, and when you eat it. As long as the food you eat is right for you (and this book is designed to help you discover which foods these are), you don't have to worry too much about the *amount* you eat.

How dieting affects muscle mass

Severe calorie restriction forces the body to use not only fat to make up for the energy deficit, but protein as well. The protein the body uses as a sort of top-up fuel comes from muscle. The real aim of any weight loss programme is to lose fat, not muscle. Muscle bulk and strength determines our capacity for physical work and exercise, so preserving it is of prime importance to health and well-being (see chapter 10, *Move It*, for information on how to preserve muscle mass using simple exercises).

Apart from their role in posture and movement, muscles are also where most of the metabolic work goes on in the body. Other tissue components, such as fat, bone and nervous tissue, do not need much in the way of fuel to keep them going. Muscle, on the other hand, is essentially the body's engine house and this is where the bulk of the body's fuel is burnt. If we lose muscle bulk our overall capacity to burn fuel declines. With this comes an inevitable decline in our ability to lose weight and an increase in the chances that we will put it on.

How dieting affects vital nutrients

The reactions that burn food for energy are dependent on the supply of certain nutrients, such as magnesium and the B vitamins. For efficient fat-burning potential, it is important that we keep up our intake of a wide range of essential nutrients. The official line put forward by some doctors is that we get everything we need from our diet, but this is simply not so. Due to poor food quality and less than healthy dietary choices, nutritional deficiencies are rife in the Western world, and can only have a negative impact on our health and well-being (3, 4).

While on a diet, food quantity generally declines. There is almost an inevitable reduction in our intake of nutrients. Bearing in mind that we need a range of nutrients for the breakdown of food and fat stores in the body, we can see that nutrient deficiency is yet another way dieting may lead us into problems.

Calorie-based diets place more emphasis on the quantity of food, rather than the quality. Even an apparently healthy diet is unlikely to supply all the vitamins and minerals we need in the amounts necessary for peak health. When we begin to cut down on the amount of food we eat, and at the same time eat foods which are low in nutrients (as most diet foods are), we are in grave danger of suffering from the effects of vitamin and mineral depletion.

Not all calories are the same

Another potential pitfall of low-calorie dieting is that there is a tendency to become focused on the calorific content of foods, rather than their health-giving potential. Using the calorie approach, the form that food comes in recedes in importance compared to the actual amount of calories the food contains. As a result, individuals can end up eating some pretty unwholesome foods, which are unlikely to enhance health in the long term. Low calorie pre-prepared meals and desserts are good examples. These foods are often highly processed, full of artificial additives and bereft of the nutrients so important to health.

This preoccupation with calories can cloud the basic issue that not all calories are the same. Calories can come in three main forms: carbohydrate, protein and fat. To lay down food as fat, the body has to put a bit of energy in. For the body to take 100 calories of fat and lay this down as fat in the tissues, 2½ calories must be expended. That's not a lot of energy because, in essence, it doesn't take much to take dietary fat and dump it as fat in the tissues. However, converting carbohydrate or protein into fat requires much more biochemical processing, and therefore more energy must be expended as a result. In fact, to convert 100 calories worth of protein or carbohydrate into fat the body needs to expend 23 calories, almost ten times the amount needed to process the equivalent amount of fat. Even if calorie intake is the same, a high-fat diet is more likely to lead to weight gain than a high-carbohydrate or high-protein diet.

Slim chance

With rates of overweight and obesity rising sharply, the food industry has been quick to cash in on this trend. The supermarket shelves are awash with products claiming to be 'diet', 'lite' and 'low fat'. It stands to reason that anyone with their heart set on losing a few surplus pounds could do worse than invest in some of the slimming and diet foods that usually promise weight loss if used 'as part of a calorie-controlled diet'. The reality is that few of these foods actually deliver on this promise, and the only place they're likely to leave you feeling lighter is in the purse or wallet.

First of all, let's look at the claim that these foods can help you lose weight as long as they're eaten in conjunction with a calorie-controlled diet. Well, one could argue that any food helps weight loss if it is part of a calorie-controlled diet, even a double serving of chocolate fudge cake with lashings of cream. The statutory claim made by many slimming products is quite meaningless.

Looking at the products themselves, how do they compare to their non-slimming counterparts? I recently took a trip around my local supermarket to see what was in store for the unsuspecting slimmer. I picked up a loaf of slimmers' bread, which boasted 'only 28 calories per slice'. Actually, weight for weight, this bread has no fewer calories than standard white bread at all. The reason that it only has 28 calories per slice is because the slices are pitifully small.

Another product I chanced upon was a slimmer's minestrone packet soup. This soup contained 59 calories per serving, while its non-slimming version contained 95 calories. Interestingly, weight for weight, the slimmer's soup actually contained more fat than its non-slimming version and their ingredients were virtually identical. So how did the manufacturer manage to reduce the calorie content of their product? By reducing the serving size from 25g to 15g, that's how. Oh, and just in case you're wondering, the pack prices were identical.

I could go on to give countless other examples, but the basic point is: slimming foods are very rarely worth the premium prices you pay for them and are unlikely to help you lose weight in the long term. It is my firm belief that it is possible to lose weight without ever having to revert to using foods marketed specifically to dieters.

Graze, don't gorge

A central theme in many weight loss regimes where calorie restriction is an integral factor is that three meals should be eaten, but snacks should be avoided in between. The principle here is that snacking between meals just ups the calorie intake for the day and therefore could not possibly help in weight loss. In fact, it turns out that just the reverse is true. Eating in between meals can actually speed weight loss because it helps to keep that fire going inside. In one study, rats were given an amount of food during a one-hour period each day. A second group of rats were given the same type and amount of food, this time divided into six feeding sessions throughout the day. The first group of rats tended to become overweight, but the second group did not. This is a very clear demonstration of the fact that grazing food throughout the day can actually help weight loss.

The benefits of grazing food go beyond improved weight loss. In another study, human volunteers were split into two groups. One group was given a certain amount and type of food as three meals over the course of a day. The other group was given exactly the same type and amount of food, but this time it was divided into 17 (yes, that's right, *seventeen*) snacks during the day (5). After only two weeks the subjects on the grazing diet had significantly lower levels of cholesterol in their bloodstream. The levels of insulin were also lower in this group, which is particularly relevant as insulin stimulates the production of fat in the body. For more about the effect of insulin in the body and how to control insulin levels, read chapter 3, *Balance Your Blood Sugar*.

Another possible reason why grazing is good for us is that it may help improve digestion. The body only has a finite capacity to digest food at any time; the larger the meal we eat, the more likely that some of this is going to end up being undigested. Undigested food can wreak havoc in the body and does nothing to contribute to weight loss and health. For more information about this, read chapter 6, *Eliminate Your Allergies*. Eating two or three large meals each day can be hard work for the digestive system. By eating smaller amounts of food more regularly, it is more likely that the digestive system will digest food fully and completely.

Eating for healthy weight loss

The fundamentals for weight loss with regard to eating patterns are:

1. Eat three meals a day

2. Eat so that you are satisfied

3. Eat healthy snacks in between meals

Now let's look at these principles in more detail:

1. Eat three meals a day

For the best weight loss and maximum health it is very important for most individuals to eat three meals a day. One of the more important meals is breakfast. This is the meal that gets your metabolism going after a whole night of being starved of fuel. Now, I've seen a lot of weight-conscious people who do not eat breakfast because they are not hungry in the morning, and besides, eating breakfast just makes them hungrier. People who are not hungry in the morning often have just got out of the habit of not eating breakfast and generally feel safe not eating it. If they're not eating they can't possibly be putting on weight, right? Well, as we've discussed, while not eating may help weight loss at that particular time, it's setting the body up for more problems later on.

If you have not eaten breakfast for some time, then I generally recommend a smallish, manageable meal to begin with. Some fresh fruit is often a good option, maybe with a bit of natural yoghurt. Or perhaps a poached egg on some wholegrain toast. A small bowl of unsweetened muesli topped with some natural yoghurt and sliced fruit is another idea.

2. Eat so that you are satisfied

One of the questions that individuals wishing to lose weight often ask is 'How much should I eat?' This preoccupation with meal size usually stems from more than a couple of scrapes with calorie-based dieting. Thinking back to the internal fire will help you decide on portion size. If you are hungry, eat until you feel satisfied and then stop. If your flames are dwindling, you'll want to put a fair amount of fuel on the fire, but you don't want to smother it either. If possible, eat slowly and savour your food. This really does cut down on your chances of eating more than your body needs at that time. If you have spent some months, or even years, suppressing feelings of hunger, it may take you a while to get back in touch with what is a healthy meal size for you. In time, though, you'll get used to what is right for you.

3. Eat healthy snacks in between meals

The idea of grazing food may seem utterly alien to you if you have tried to restrict calories in the past, but this should not detract from the fact that there are sound physiological reasons for eating to this pattern. As a general rule, I recommend fruit as the ideal between-meal snack. Most fresh fruits release sugar quite slowly into the bloodstream (the significance of this is explained in chapter 3, *Balance Your Blood Sugar*). Fruit is also relatively easy to digest and therefore gives us fuel without overwhelming our internal fire. Fruit is also convenient as it takes little or no preparation and can usually be found without too much effort. And, finally, fruit is nutritious. High in fibre and essential nutrients, adding fruit between meals is an ideal way to upgrade the general quality of the diet.

Case Study

Mary G is a 36-year-old legal secretary

About 18 months ago I was hovering just under the 10 stone mark. At 5' 4" I was not dramatically overweight, I know, but I was really not comfortable with myself. I remember having this dream of getting down to 9 stones, the weight I was when I was 20 years old. Ever since, I had battled with my weight. I had started endless diets and had not been able to stick to any of them. My weight had gradually crept up over the years.

Over the last couple of years I had settled on an eating plan which allowed me to at least maintain, if not lose, weight. I ate half a grapefruit and half a slice of brown toast in the morning, a plain tuna or chicken sandwich at lunch and a small piece of fish with vegetables (no potatoes) in the evening. I was almost permanently hungry on this regime. However, if I deviated from it, boy, would I pay! A meal out or take-away could put on two or three pounds that would take several weeks to work off.

I obsessively counted calories – everything I thought about eating was first reduced to its calorific value. Then I finally decided it was time to get out and find some way of managing my weight without the need to count calories or be perpetually hungry. I decided to seek some professional advice and ended up consulting a nutritionist.

My practitioner explained to me about the effect long-term dieting could have on the metabolism. My ideas about calories were very entrenched, but he very patiently broke down these views. We decided that I should take a very simple approach to my weight problem. To begin with, breakfast was to be more of an event – a good-sized fresh fruit salad with some live natural yoghurt. I added a salad to my sandwich at lunch and changed the bread from white to wholemeal. The evening meal was kept the same, but with no restriction on volume. Another change I made was in my pattern of eating – instead of eating three meals a day, I started to graze food, eating a piece of fruit between breakfast and lunch and lunch and supper.

During the first two weeks on this programme, my weight did not change at all. However, the way I reasoned it was that if I was less hungry and not putting on weight, it had to be a good thing. Also, because I was eating more healthily, my general levels of energy and vitality improved. I was becoming more confident with my eating and was definitely coming round to the idea that eating more did not necessarily mean putting on weight.

After the initial two weeks, I was thrilled to find that I had started to lose weight. It was nothing dramatic. I think I lost about a pound every two weeks. At the end of six months though I had lost 12 pounds. I was down to what I considered to be a healthy weight for me and was no longer having to starve myself. I had learnt a whole new way of looking at food which really worked.

Summary

- Restricting calories can reduce the body's ability to burn food, may cause the body to lose muscle tissue and is likely to contribute to nutritional deficiencies in the long term.

- Eating stimulates the metabolism and can therefore contribute to weight loss in the long term.

- To achieve continued weight loss, it is important to eat three meals a day.

- Healthy snacks such as fruit should be taken in between meals.

- Remember, the secret to losing weight for many people is not to eat *less*, but to eat *more*.

CHAPTER 3

Balance Your Blood Sugar

Do you sometimes crave sweet or starchy foods? Find that you feel tired and unable to concentrate in the mid- to late afternoon? Can you become irritable or shaky if you skip a meal? Do you wake up feeling tired and groggy in the morning, even after a good night's sleep? If you've answered 'yes' to any of these questions, then there's a better than even chance that the level of sugar in your bloodstream tends to fluctuate abnormally. This problem, often referred to as 'hypoglycaemia' or 'impaired glucose tolerance', is a common and generally unrecognized cause of excess weight. What is more, if left untreated, it may lead to significant health problems in the long term, including heart disease and diabetes. The good news is that with a few simple changes to your diet and some well-chosen nutritional supplements, it is possible to stabilize blood-sugar levels and take control of your weight, and your health, in the long term.

The body in balance

Every moment of every day, the body adjusts its internal mechanisms to keep it in balance. For instance, if thyroid function declines for any reason, the body makes a hormone that tells the thyroid to work harder. If the temperature around us rises, sweating increases and the blood vessels in the skin dilate in an effort to keep cool. The name given to this principle of internal balance is 'homeostasis'.

One very important component of homeostasis is the regulation of the level of sugar in the bloodstream. For a significant proportion of the population, the mechanisms designed to keep blood-sugar levels on an even keel may fail, and this very often leads to problems with weight gain and ill-health. Before we discuss what can go wrong, let's take a look at how it's supposed to be.

Blood-sugar balance and health

For most of us, a significant proportion of our diet comes in the form of carbohydrates such as sugars (e.g. fruit, fruit juices, confectionery, cake, biscuits and desserts) and starches (e.g. bread, potatoes, rice and pasta). Starches actually consist of very long chains of sugar molecules, which are too long to be absorbed through the gut and into the bloodstream. Consequently, in order to absorb starches, we must first break them down into their single sugar components through the processes of digestion.

Whether we eat sugars or starches, a rise in the sugar level of the bloodstream occurs. As blood-sugar levels rise, the pancreas secretes a hormone called insulin. One of the chief effects of insulin is to transport sugar out of the bloodstream and into the body's cells. In this way, blood-sugar levels are lowered, preventing the accumulation of sugar in the bloodstream.

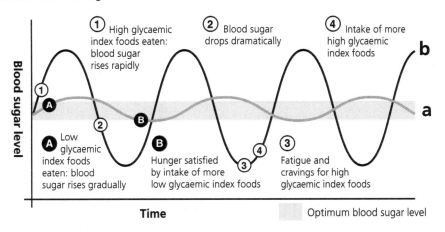

In an ideal world, the body likes to keep the level of sugar within relatively narrow parameters. It helps the body to get its fuel from foods that release sugar slowly into the bloodstream. Controlled, sustained releases of sugar into the bloodstream allow the body to keep sugar levels in balance (see diagram above line, **a**).

However, if the blood-sugar levels rise very quickly, the body has to secrete a lot of insulin in response. While this may well be effective in bringing the blood-sugar level down to normal, it may also lead to low levels of blood sugar as the body over-compensates for the initial rise (see diagram above, line **b**). Low blood sugar (hypoglycaemia) can induce some pretty unwelcome symptoms. These include:

1. Fatigue

Sugar is *the* main fuel in the body. If the level of sugar in the blood drops, fatigue is inevitable. We may have good stores of energy in the form of fat or glycogen (a form of starch in the muscles and liver), but if the sugar concentration in the blood is inadequate, the body's engine is likely to stall. Low blood sugar is a bit like having a full tank of petrol with none of it getting through to the engine.

2. The mid-afternoon slump

A classic time for the fatigue associated with hypoglycaemia is the mid- to late afternoon. This effect is caused essentially by the body's reaction to lunch. The big rise in blood sugar that often follows this meal can trigger a huge insulin surge, leading to low blood sugar later on. A blood-sugar problem is usually the cause of the mid- to late afternoon crash some people experience.

3. Morning grogginess

The fatigue associated with hypoglycaemia is often at its worst first thing in the morning because hypoglycaemics tend not to maintain blood-sugar levels when they are asleep. Those who feel tired and groggy in the morning, even after eight or more hours of decent sleep, often have a problem with hypoglycaemia.

4. Mood disturbance

For an organ which only accounts for about 2% of our weight, the brain sure does use a lot of sugar. At rest, the brain uses about half the sugar circulating in our bloodstream. What's more, while most of the body can use other foods to generate energy, the brain is almost entirely reliant on sugar as a fuel. If the sugar level drops in the brain, then the brain doesn't work so well; it's as simple as that. Common mental manifestations of this include poor concentration, memory lapses, depression, irritability and mood swings.

5. Waking in the night

When blood-sugar levels drop during the night, the body will normally take steps to maintain balance. It does this by secreting hormones, which have a blood-sugar raising effect, especially adrenaline. Adrenaline is the hormone we make when we're under stress and it generally promotes feelings of anxiety and alertness. Not the ideal hormone to have whooshing around our bloodstream in the middle of the night. Blood-sugar problems are a very common cause of sleep disruption.

6. Food cravings

Another common symptom of hypoglycaemia is food cravings. If our blood-sugar levels drop, it is natural for our body to crave foods it knows will restore the blood-sugar levels quickly. That's why some of us crave sweet or starchy foods from time to time. For many women, food cravings tend to be worse just before a period, as hormonal fluctuations at this time can disrupt the blood-sugar balance.

Is blood-sugar imbalance your problem?

This questionnaire is designed to help you assess whether blood-sugar imbalance is a factor in you. Score each question as indicated and then add up your total score.

1. Does your energy tend to fluctuate during the day?
No –   0 points
Occasional or mild symptoms –   2 points
Frequent or severe problems –   4 points

2. Do you find that eating something can often pick up your energy level?
No –   0 points
Occasionally –   2 points
Frequently –   4 points

3. Do you often feel tired or unable to concentrate in the mid- or late afternoon?
No –   0 points
Occasional or mild problems –   2 points
Frequent or severe problems –   4 points

4. Do you feel tired or groggy on waking, despite sleeping for eight or more hours?
No –   0 points
Occasional or mild problems –   2 points
Frequent or severe problems –   4 points

5. Do you tend to wake in the middle of the night, sometimes feeling anxious or nervy?

No –	0 points
Occasional or mild problems –	3 points
Frequent or severe problems –	5 points

6. Are you prone to mood swings and/or irritability, especially if a meal is skipped?

No –	0 points
Occasional or mild problems –	2 points
Frequent or severe problems –	4 points

7. Can you crave sweet or starchy foods from time to time?

No –	0 points
Occasional or mild symptoms –	3 points
Frequent or severe symptoms –	5 points

8. Do you feel you need to eat very regularly?

No –	0 points
Occasional or mild problems –	2 points
Frequent or severe problems –	4 points

9. Do you find yourself craving alcohol in the early evening?

No –	0 points
Occasional or mild problems –	1 points
Frequent or severe problems –	2 points

10. Do you have a history of Type II (mature-onset) diabetes in your family? (see page 45)

No –	0 points
Yes –	4 points

Interpreting your score

0 – 9:	blood-sugar imbalance is unlikely
10 – 19:	blood-sugar imbalance is quite likely and measures taken to stabilize blood sugar could be of benefit
20 and above:	blood-sugar imbalance is likely, and measures taken to stabilize blood sugar are highly recommended

Blood tests for blood-sugar balance

The symptoms of impaired blood-sugar balance are usually clear-cut enough to enable a diagnosis to be made without the need for testing. However, tests are available, and their relative merits are discussed here:

The Random Blood Glucose Test

The most commonly performed test for hypoglycaemia is the Random Blood Glucose Test. Here, a sample of blood is drawn and analyzed for its glucose (sugar) concentration. However, this test only provides a snapshot in time of the level of sugar in the bloodstream. As blood-sugar levels can vary greatly during the day, this test is virtually useless for the assessment of blood sugar stability.

The Glucose Tolerance Test

A more useful test in the diagnosis of blood-sugar imbalance is the Glucose Tolerance Test (GTT). Here, a sample of blood is drawn, after which 50g of glucose is administered to the test subject in the form of a sugary drink. Blood samples, usually taken at hourly intervals for five hours, are then analyzed for glucose. In individuals who have a problem regulating blood sugar, the test may reveal a rapid rise in blood sugar that often peaks at a level higher than we would like. In addition, this initial rise is often followed by a lower than normal blood sugar some time later. While it has its place, some doctors and scientists believe that even the GTT is not the best test for blood-sugar imbalance (1). It is now thought that measuring insulin levels during the GTT is critical to the accuracy of this test. This test, known as the Glucose-Insulin Tolerance Test (see below), is increasingly regarded as the most relevant test for blood-sugar imbalance.

The Glucose-Insulin Tolerance Test

In a Glucose-Insulin Tolerance Test (GITT), insulin levels are measured with sugar levels for up to five hours. This test may reveal elevated insulin levels in subjects who have normal blood-sugar levels (2). Because of this, the GITT is thought to be a much more sensitive indicator of blood-sugar balance than the GTT.

The GITT can be a very useful test because of its ability to pick up elevated insulin levels. While insulin is essential to life, we can get too much of a good thing.

The effects of excess insulin

Some of the effects of excess insulin include:

1. Fat production

Insulin stimulates the conversion of sugar into a starch-like substance called glycogen in the liver and muscle. However, when the glycogen stores in the body are full, insulin stimulates the production of substances called triglycerides, which is fancy language for fat. In other words, the body takes the excess sugar in the bloodstream and converts a proportion of it into fat. People with blood-sugar imbalance tend to put on weight for this reason.

2. Fat around the middle

Insulin does not just cause us to accumulate weight as fat, it can also determine where that fat is deposited in the body. In general terms, fat can either be deposited around the middle (so-called 'abdominal' fat) producing a rounded, apple-shaped appearance to the body, or below the waist (also known as 'gluteal' fat), giving the body a pear-shaped appearance. Abdominal fat seems to be a much better predictor of certain diseases than gluteal fat. Abdominal fat appears to increase the risk of serious conditions such as heart disease, high blood pressure, high levels of cholesterol in the blood, diabetes and certain forms of cancer. Another bad bit of news about insulin is that its presence tends to favour the accumulation of abdominal rather than gluteal fat.

3. High blood pressure and fluid retention

Many of the mechanisms the body uses to balance the amount of fluid it contains, along with the levels of key substances such as sodium, potassium and chloride, take place in the kidneys. In the kidneys, insulin causes the body to hang on to sodium (sodium retention) and, in time, this can predispose to high blood pressure (hypertension) and fluid retention.

4. Raised cholesterol

Insulin stimulates the liver to make more of an enzyme called HMG-CoA reductase. The function of this enzyme is to manufacture cholesterol, raising levels of this substance in the bloodstream. The higher the level of cholesterol in the bloodstream, the greater the risk of heart disease and stroke.

5. Symptoms of hypoglycaemia

There is some evidence that the symptoms of hypoglycaemia, such as fatigue and anxiety, may actually be related to high levels of insulin in the bloodstream, irrespective of the blood-sugar level. Also, the symptoms of hypoglycaemia seem to come on at higher levels of blood sugar, when insulin levels are high.

6. Type II diabetes

High levels of insulin in the body can increase the risk of diabetes. If the body secretes a lot of insulin over many years, then it can become increasingly less sensitive to the effect of that insulin. This may lead to a condition known as Type II diabetes (also known as mature onset or non-insulin dependent diabetes). This normally comes on in middle or old age and makes up about 85% of all diabetic cases. Sufferers of this form of diabetes may be able to control their diabetes through changing their diet. If this fails, oral medication may be prescribed. A proportion of Type II diabetics may need insulin to control their condition. Many doctors and scientists are reaching the conclusion that the more out of balance our blood-sugar level is, the more insulin we secrete and the more likely we are to become resistant to its effects. Taking steps to improve blood-sugar control is likely to reduce your risk of developing diabetes in the long term.

The bottom line

Blood-sugar fluctuation can have disastrous consequences for the would-be slimmer. High levels of sugar in the bloodstream lead to the over-production of insulin, which increases the storage of fat in the body and can also cause the body to retain fluid. Low blood-sugar levels tend to cause us to crave unhealthy, sugar-laden foods such as chocolate, cakes, sugared breakfast cereals and soft drinks. Plus, the frequent bouts of fatigue that are common with hypoglycaemia make exercise a real non-event for many sufferers. If you want to lose weight and believe that blood-sugar imbalance is part of your picture, gaining control is top priority for you. Here's how:

The GI Scale and healthy food choices

One important factor in getting blood sugar back in balance is to eat a diet based on foods that give a controlled release of sugar into the body. The speed and extent to which a food increases blood sugar can be quantified using the Glycaemic Index (GI) Scale. The higher a food's glycaemic index, the faster it releases sugar into the bloodstream. A food's glycaemic index is related to a variety of factors, including the principle form of sugar it contains and its fibre content.

Sugar type

There are three principal sugars that make up carbohydrates: glucose, fructose and galactose. Glucose is the main sugar in sweet foods (other than fruit), vegetables and grains such as wheat, oats, rye and rice. Fructose is the sugar found in fruit, while galactose is found in dairy products, principally milk. Once sugar has been absorbed from the gut, it travels directly to the liver. Glucose needs no processing before it can be passed into the bloodstream proper. As a result, foods that contain glucose have the capacity to bring about very rapid rises in blood sugar.

Unlike glucose, both fructose and galactose need to be processed in the liver before they can be released into the bloodstream as glucose. As a result of this process, foods which contain these sugars generally give slow, sustained releases of sugar into the bloodstream.

Fibre

Fibre is not absorbed from food and therefore does not have any direct effect on blood sugar or insulin levels. However, the more fibre there is in food, the more slowly sugars are released from it, and the lower the glycaemic index. Thus, unrefined, whole starches such as wholemeal bread and brown rice, will tend to have lower glycaemic indices than their refined counterparts.

Common Foods and their Glycaemic Indices

The following lists give a rank order of the commonly eaten carbohydrate foods and their glycaemic indices. In this scheme, glucose (the fastest releasing foodstuff) is given an arbitrary value of 100, and all other foods are compared to this.

High Glycaemic Index Foods (fast-releasing foods)		Low Glycaemic Index Foods (slow-releasing foods)	
glucose	100	brown rice	50
baked potatoes	95	wholemeal bread	50
honey	90	wholewheat pasta	45
white bread	85	oats	40
cornflakes	85	whole rye bread	40
carrots, cooked	85	peas	40
sugar	75	unsweetened fresh fruit juice	40
sugared breakfast cereal	70	whole cereals	35
chocolate bars	70	fresh fruit	35
sweetcorn	70	lentils	30
white rice	70	chick peas	30
boiled potatoes	70	green vegetables	less than 15
non-wholewheat pasta	65	tomatoes	less than 15
bananas	60	mushrooms	less than 15
dried fruit	60		
jam	55		

Keeping your diet weighted towards unrefined starches such as wholemeal (wholewheat) bread, wholewheat pasta and brown rice, beans, pulses, fresh fruits and vegetables, will help to maintain blood-sugar stability and help you lose weight, too. A bit later in this chapter there will be some meal suggestions designed specifically for blood-sugar control.

Some fast-releasing food may be OK

You might be wondering if you need to completely exclude the high glycaemic index foods from your diet. The answer is, no, not necessarily. While the glycaemic index scores are a good guide to the tendency of a food to upset blood sugar, they actually represent the effect of a standard amount of that food eaten on its own. Basically, if we eat a lot of a high glycaemic index food, the chances are we'll experience a massive rise in blood sugar and a huge surge of insulin to go with it. A much smaller amount of the same food is obviously going to be much less disruptive to the system. There's a world of difference, therefore, between eating a huge baked potato and a small handful of chips or crisps.

Another way of eating high glycaemic index foods, and increasing our chances of getting away with it, is to mix them with foods which release sugar more slowly into the bloodstream. The fibre and other dietary elements in some foods appear to delay the release of sugar from other foods when eaten with them. Let's say, for instance, that you're going to eat a meal that contains white rice. If you eat the white rice on its own, you'll almost certainly be in for trouble. However, if that white rice is eaten as part of a meal which also contains a chicken dish and some fresh, steamed vegetables, it is much more likely that there will be a controlled release of sugar into the bloodstream.

Regular meals for hypoglycaemics

The majority of hypoglycaemics do not maintain blood-sugar levels at all well if a meal is skipped or delayed significantly. It makes sense, therefore, for anyone whose blood sugar tends to run a bit on the low side to have meals at regular intervals. As a general rule, breakfast, lunch and dinner should be the cornerstones of the hypoglycaemic's eating regime. However, at least in the initial stages of re-establishing better blood-sugar control, it is almost always beneficial for healthy snacks to be had between meals, too.

The afternoon is usually a real danger time for most hypoglycaemics. The insulin surge that comes after lunch can drive blood-sugar levels down in the mid- to late afternoon. The chances are you'll have experienced this and will be all too familiar with the feelings of lethargy, drowsiness and foggy brain at this time. Another common manifestation of the afternoon slump is a desire to eat or drink a 'little something'. This little something, be it a cake, biscuit or soft drink, will almost certainly send the blood sugar sky-rocketing again. This might get you out of a tight spot for the next hour or so, but there's a pretty good chance the blood sugar will come crashing down again, leaving you at square one.

Tactical eating

To get over the afternoon blues, it can be useful to employ the principle of tactical eating. What this means is having something to eat in anticipation of low blood sugar later on, even if you don't feel hungry. Now, I know this goes against the grain of that standard tenet in dieting, which states that you should never eat when you're not hungry. However, the problem is that hypoglycaemia does tend to creep up on us. One moment we can be cruising through the afternoon full of beans, the next we can be yawning and reaching for the biscuits. If you're trying to get your blood-sugar level back on an even keel, it can be very beneficial for you to pre-empt this classic scenario. Eating something before your blood-sugar level drops into your boots can stop the problem in its tracks. So, if you tend to fall to bits at around 4.00pm, why not eat a piece or two of fruit at around 3.00pm? It could really save you a lot of grief later in the day.

A snack before bedtime

If you have a tendency towards hypoglycaemia, another good time for you to eat is before bed. Now, I know you've read that eating before you go to sleep is not good because the digestion slows down in the evening and this can lead to problems with indigestion and disturbed sleep. I agree with this general principle. However, remember that many hypoglycaemics fail to maintain blood-sugar levels overnight, and this can lead to insomnia and morning fatigue. Remember, also, that if the blood-sugar level falls as we sleep, the body secretes hormones such as adrenaline, which can disturb the quality and amount of sleep we get.

Apart from putting into practice the general advice here about controlling blood sugar, it could also benefit you to eat a snack before you go to bed. Giving your body a bit of fuel 'to chew on' while you sleep may be all it takes to maintain your blood-sugar level at night. With less need to have adrenaline coursing through your body, the chances are you'll sleep much more soundly. Another welcome spin-off is that you might actually feel vaguely human in the morning.

Protein and blood-sugar control

We know that insulin lowers blood-sugar levels. However, there is another important hormone called glucagon, which has the opposite effect. Also secreted by the pancreas, glucagon works in concert with insulin, balancing its effect. You could argue that low blood sugar is not just a result of excessive insulin production but inadequate glucagon production, too. In other words, if we can get the body to produce more glucagon, maybe that will help stabilize blood-sugar levels. Well, it turns out that one of the major triggers for the release of glucagon is dietary protein, and it has been suggested that in addition to cutting back on fast-releasing carbohydrates, we should be upping our intake of protein, too. This theory is a central theme in the book entitled *The Zone* by Dr Barry Sears. I have to say, I have found the addition of significant amounts of protein in the diets of my hypoglycaemic clients to be very beneficial in the great majority of cases. The question is, how much protein should you add?

Well, the answer is that it's not so much the amount of protein, but the protein-to-carbohydrate ratio that seems to be important here. If you want to get into the nitty-gritty of this and feel compelled to start calculating the protein and carbohydrate contents of some of your favourite foods, you'd better invest in a copy of *The Zone*. If, however, you want a simple, low-tech guide to using protein to balance your blood sugar, then you really need to know only two things:

1. If you are eating fast-releasing carbohydrate (white bread, white rice, white pasta, potato) then you need approximately the same volume of protein (meat, fish, egg, tofu) to maintain blood-sugar levels. In other words, if you are eating a small baked potato you're going to need a leg of chicken or a whole 7 oz (200 g) can of tuna to balance this.

2. If you are eating slow-releasing carbohydrate (brown rice, wholemeal bread, wholewheat pasta) then you need about half as much in the way of protein to keep your blood sugar on an even keel.

To these meals you can add all the green and leafy vegetables you want.

Caffeine and blood-sugar control

Two of the favourite props used by hypoglycaemics who are trying to lose weight are black coffee and diet cola drinks. These are virtually devoid of calories and pretty much guaranteed to pick up energy levels while staving off hunger, what could be better? Well, you're not going to like this, but caffeinated drinks, such as coffee and diet cola, are a bit of a disaster for hypoglycaemics. The reason is that caffeine stimulates the secretion of insulin, effectively destabilizing the blood-sugar system. Caffeine, because it has stimulant effects on the body, will almost certainly pick up flagging energy levels in the short term but its effect on blood sugar generally leads to a huge slump in energy later on.

Another downside to the consumption of caffeine is that it appears to worsen the symptoms of hypoglycaemia. This means that for a given level of blood sugar, hypoglycaemic symptoms are more likely and generally more pronounced if there is caffeine in the system.

Coming off caffeine

If you habitually take caffeine in your diet, either in coffee, tea or caffeinated soft drinks, then you would do well to kick, or at least moderate, this habit. One way to get off caffeine is the 'cold turkey' method, which means just stopping caffeine intake dead. This method is quick, but there's usually a price to pay. Anyone with a half-decent caffeine intake is likely to get caffeine-withdrawal symptoms, which normally manifest themselves as general fatigue accompanied by a horrendous headache. These symptoms usually last a couple of days, after which a state of calm returns pretty briskly to the system. Another way of coming off caffeine is to gradually reduce your intake. This takes longer than the cold turkey method the effects are much less painful.

I generally advise my clients to reduce their intake of caffeine by a drink per day every three or four days. This means that if they drink five cups of coffee a day, for three or four days they should drink four cups per day, reducing this to three cups per day and so on until they're drinking nothing at all. Another tactic is to swap caffeinated drinks for decaffeinated versions. Look out for coffee which has been decaffeinated using the water or 'Swiss' method. This method of decaffeination avoids the potentially hazardous substances which are sometimes used in the extraction process.

Artificial sweeteners

Many individuals may look forward to reducing their intake of sugar with some trepidation. The natural tendency may be to opt for artificial sweeteners instead.

However, there is emerging evidence that sweeteners such as aspartame and saccharin are not necessarily the healthy alternatives to sugar that they're made out to be. Aspartame may reduce levels of the brain chemical serotonin, which in turn can lead to mood and sleep disturbances (3). Large amounts of aspartame may provoke headaches, fainting, seizures, memory loss, mood swings, depression and nausea. Small doses can cause itching and rashes in susceptible individuals.

And, if that isn't enough, there is some scientific evidence to suggest that artificial sweeteners may actually encourage us to eat more in the long term (4). In one study researchers found that subjects were inclined to eat more after eating yoghurt sweetened with saccharin than those who had eaten yoghurt sweetened with sugar (5). One study showed that saccharin induced hypoglycaemia in test subjects, even if it was only tasted and not swallowed (6). It looks as though the body just can't be fooled into feeling satisfied by mimicking more natural sources of sweetness.

Before you think I'm sounding mean and miserable about this, let me tell you that there is a natural sweetener that I think can be used quite safely by hypoglycaemics. It's called Stevia, and is an extract of a tree native to South America. Stevia has been used for centuries by traditional South American cultures as a sweetening agent and is very popular in Japan. It can be added to hot beverages or used in baking. Because only very small amounts of Stevia need to be used to get a sweetening effect, it is also very economical. You can find it in powder and liquid form in health-foods stores. Alternatively, to obtain Stevia by mail order, look in the section entitled 'Useful Information' at the end of the book, under the name *Rio Trading*.

Menu suggestions for stabilizing blood-sugar levels

With the theory behind us, what does all this mean in practical terms? Here are some meal ideas based on the fundamental principles outlined in this chapter:

Breakfast

Poached egg on whole-rye toast with grilled tomato

Poached or grilled haddock or kipper with grilled tomato, mushrooms and wholewheat or whole-rye toast

Unsweetened muesli with milk (cow's, goat's, rice, soya), live natural yoghurt, seeds and fresh fruit

Oat porridge (oatmeal) made with banana, topped with live natural yoghurt

Lunch/Dinner

Grilled trout or chicken with fresh steamed vegetables and a few boiled new potatoes

Brown rice salad made with chicken or fish, chopped vegetables (e.g. tomato, cucumber), beans and pulses

Spanish omelette with salad

Chicken, tuna or salmon salad sandwich on wholemeal or whole-rye bread

Wholewheat pasta with meat or fish sauce and salad

Chicken or fish with brown rice and steamed vegetables.

In-between-meal snacks

Raw nuts and seeds

Fresh fruit

Rye cracker with chicken and tomato topping

Nutrients for blood-sugar balance

The processes that regulate the level of sugar in the bloodstream are dependent on hormones and enzymes. The function of these hormones and enzymes is, at least in part, dependent on the availability of certain nutrients. What follows is a guide to the most important nutrients that can help to combat hypoglycaemia and return you to a state of well-being.

Chromium polynicotinate – the trace mineral chromium has a very important part to play in the regulation of blood-sugar levels, and can be effective in combating hypoglycaemia (7,8). It seems to have the capacity to regulate the action of insulin in the body, and in so doing helps in ensuring the efficient handling and metabolism of sugar. There are two commonly available forms of chromium – picolinate and polynicotinate. The polynicotinate form is closer in structure to the form of chromium found naturally in the body, something known as Glucose Tolerance Factor Chromium.

Manganese – this trace mineral plays an important part in activating the enzymes involved in sugar metabolism in the body (9).

Magnesium – this mineral is very important for blood-sugar regulation. One of its key actions is to activate the enzymes which mediate the conversion of glycogen (a storage carbohydrate) in the body to sugar, and vice versa. Magnesium supplementation has been shown to improve the action of insulin and stabilize the blood-sugar levels (10).

There are several different forms of magnesium available. Some of the most useful forms for blood-sugar balance include:

> **Magnesium ascorbate** – actually a buffered form of vitamin C, this nutrient can also help support adrenal gland function, which is often weakened in cases of sugar dysregulation.

> **Magnesium pantothenate** – also known as vitamin B5, this nutrient also supports adrenal gland function.

> **Magnesium malate and magnesium fumarate** – even if glucose levels are adequate, it is important that the body is able to actually metabolize this sugar to generate energy. The metabolism of sugar in the body is mediated through a system of biochemical reactions known as the Kreb's cycle. Magnesium malate and magnesium fumarate are good sources of malic acid and fumaric acid respectively. As they feed the Kreb's cycle they can therefore improve energy production in the body.

Vitamins B1, B2 and B3 – all of these nutrients have a critical role to play in the metabolism of carbohydrate sources of energy in the body. Vitamin B3 (niacin) is particularly important for blood sugar control, and it works with chromium to help insulin do its job in the body.

Suggested supplements

Glucoguard – a supplement specifically formulated to improve blood-sugar stability. Its chief ingredients are chromium polynicotinate, magnesium (in ascorbate, malate, fumarate and pantothenate forms), vitamins B1, B2 and B3 and manganese. For individuals who suffer from blood-sugar imbalance, regular supplementation with Glucoguard is very likely to help improve energy levels, enhance mental function and reduce the tendency for food cravings.

Contraindications

Glucoguard is not to be used in individuals with diabetes, unless under medical supervision.

Availability

Details of how to obtain Glucoguard can be found in the 'Useful Information' section at the back of the book under the name *VitaTech*.

Glutamine – this is an amino acid (a basic building block in protein). Glutamine can be used as fuel for the brain, and can therefore be very effective in reducing the carbohydrate cravings caused by hypoglycaemia. This supplement is useful in the initial stages of the rebalancing process when food cravings are likely to strike.

Recommended dosage

500–1000 mg, three or four times a day

Availability

Glutamine is widely available in health-food stores.

Case Study

Joseph K is a 56-year-old information technology manager for an accountancy firm.

> *I have always been fit and active and had never had a problem keeping my weight under control until the last ten years or so. A few pounds started creeping on, so I did the sensible thing and started watching the amount of fat in my diet. This seemed to help, but it became increasingly*

difficult to control my weight. I ended up eating virtually no fat, and filled up on carbohydrates instead. I remember I would go out with friends for dinner and stare longingly at the juicy steaks they would tuck into. I would just sit there with my pasta, feeling deprived. Despite all this self-control, I was still accumulating weight and last year tipped the scales at 14 stones, a good 25 pounds heavier than my fighting weight.

One day, while on a training course, I met a guy who had lost a lot of weight by limiting the amount of carbohydrate in his diet. Like me, he had experienced weight problems on a diet full of carbohydrates and very little fat. I had nothing to lose (except my excess baggage!) so I decided to give it a try. I began by eating eggs for breakfast, followed by meat or fish with vegetables for lunch and dinner. Some of the time I'd have a couple of potatoes or maybe some rice or pasta, but usually I'd go without. The results were dramatic. I lost 15 pounds in the first month, without ever feeling hungry. Over the next two months I lost another 8 pounds and felt very happy with my size. There were other benefits, too. I definitely have more energy now and don't seem to need so much food to keep me going. It's so weird; I wouldn't have believed that all those carbohydrates I was eating were proving to be such a problem.

Summary

- The body likes to keep the level of sugar in the bloodstream within relatively narrow limits.

- Blood-sugar instability is a major contributing factor to the problem of excess weight and other health issues, including fatigue and diabetes.

- In most cases, blood-sugar instability can be diagnosed on the basis of symptoms. The best laboratory test is the glucose insulin tolerance test.

- Individuals who suffer from blood-sugar instability should base their diet around foods which release sugar slowly into the bloodstream including wholegrains, beans, pulses, fresh fruit and vegetables (other than the potato). Protein in the diet in the form of natural yoghurt, eggs, meat, fish and tofu can also help to stabilize blood sugar levels..

- Regular meals should be taken (including breakfast) with healthy snacks, such as fruit, in between.

- Supplements of certain nutrients such as chromium, vitamin B3 and magnesium, can help improve blood-sugar stability and control the symptoms of hypoglycaemia.

- Balancing blood-sugar levels can be an effective strategy for weight loss and improved vitality.

CHAPTER 4

Keep Up the Heat

Do you tend to feel the cold and suffer from cold hands and feet? Can you find that your energy can be low for no obvious reason and that your powers of concentration and memory are not what they were? Have you been steadily putting on weight for some time, despite not having made any major changes in your eating habits or exercise regime? To be honest, do you find it very difficult to shed those extra pounds, despite doing the right things such as eating sensibly and taking more exercise? If you identify with some or all of these scenarios, then you would do well to consider the role of your thyroid gland in your weight issue.

The body's thermostat

The thyroid is a gland, about the size and shape of a bow tie, which sits in the front of the neck just above the top of the breastbone and collarbones *(see diagram opposite)*. The thyroid is essentially the body's thermostat, determining its temperature and the speed at which it burns fuel. Each cell in the body burns fuel for energy, some of which is released as heat. The speed at which the cells do this is known as the 'metabolism', and this is regulated by the thyroid gland. Bearing in mind that metabolism basically dictates the speed at which the body burns food, it won't come as much of a surprise to learn that it's a major determining factor in weight, too. If the thyroid and the metabolism are flagging, even slightly, this can lead to real problems with excess weight.

The physiology of the thyroid

The thyroid produces a variety of hormones, the most important of which is thyroxine (also known as T4). Outside the thyroid, T4 is converted into T3

Thyroid physiology

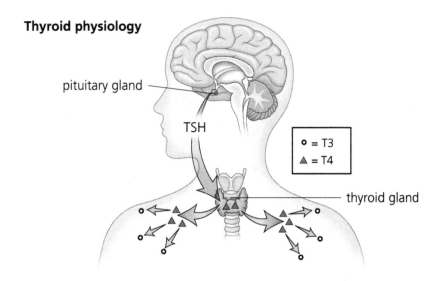

pituitary gland

TSH

○ = T3
▲ = T4

thyroid gland

(tri-iodothyronine), which is the active form of the hormone. In normal circumstances, T3 travels in the bloodstream to all the body's tissues, entering each of the body's cells. T3 stimulates cells to burn fuel with oxygen to release energy, some of this being released as heat. Essentially, the more T3 there is around, the faster the metabolism works, resulting in a reduced tendency for weight gain and a warmer body.

The thyroid's production of hormones is itself regulated by another gland, the pituitary, which sits underneath the front of the brain. One of the pituitary's jobs is to monitor and control the level of thyroid hormones in the blood. If the pituitary senses that thyroid hormone levels are dropping, it increases its own production of a substance known as thyroid stimulating hormone (TSH). This hormone instructs the thyroid to produce more thyroid hormones, thereby up-regulating the metabolism. As the thyroid-hormone levels rise, the production of TSH is down-regulated, bringing thyroid-hormone levels back down again. This mechanism is designed to ensure stable levels of thyroid hormones in the body.

The thyroid and health

The effect of the thyroid hormones on the body is far-reaching. A lack of thyroid hormones, referred to by the medical profession as hypothyroidism, can bring about a whole host of symptoms and conditions. We have already touched on the tendency for a sluggish thyroid to lead to weight gain, but, in addition, low levels of thyroid hormones in the body tend to result in the retention of water, salt and protein in the body. Blood cholesterol levels also tend to rise when thyroid hormones are deficient. The growth of the skin, hair and nails all tend to be slower when thyroid hormones are in short supply. Thyroid hormones are essential for the normal functioning of the nervous system, and mental fatigue and sluggishness are common in individuals who suffer from low thyroid function. The function of the thyroid gland is intimately interwoven with other elements of the hormone system, such as the hormone glands that control sexual function. As a result, men often manifest low thyroid function as impotence, while women may suffer from menstrual problems, such as heavy or irregular periods.

The thyroid gland and weight

Let's take a look at the relationship between thyroid function and weight in some depth. As we know, the reduced metabolism caused by a sluggish thyroid is quite likely to cause a problem with excess weight. Studies suggest that about two-thirds of individuals with low thyroid function have a weight problem. In my experience, a high percentage of overweight individuals have good evidence of hypothyroidism. For many of these individuals, the problem is not only one of weight gain, but one of a real inability to lose weight. When I see an individual who tells me that he or she just cannot seem to lose significant amounts of weight, despite cutting back on food and taking regular exercise, one of the first things I will want to explore is thyroid function. Very rarely do I see a client who finds losing weight virtually impossible and who does not have some evidence of a malfunctioning thyroid.

Is low thyroid function your problem?

The following questionnaire is designed to help you identify a potential thyroid problem. Score each question as indicated and then add up your total score.

Do you:
1. Suffer from unexplained fatigue or lethargy?

No –	0 points
Occasional or mild problems –	2 points
Frequent or severe problems –	4 points

2. Find that your energy can be low in the morning even after a good night's sleep?

No –	0 points
Occasional or mild problems –	3 points
Frequent or severe problems –	5 points

3. Feel the cold, and have to wrap up more than others?

No –	0 points
Occasional or mild problems –	3 points
Frequent or severe problems –	5 points

4. Suffer from cold hands and feet?

No –	0 points
Occasional or mild problems –	2 points
Frequent or severe problems –	4 points

5. Suffer from dry skin?

No –	0 points
Occasional or mild problems –	1 points
Frequent or severe problems –	2 points

6. Suffer from dry or brittle hair?

No –	0 points
Occasional or mild problems –	2 points
Frequent or severe problems –	4 points

7. Find that you do not sweat much, even when you exercise?

No –	0 points
Yes –	4 points

8. Suffer from constipation?

No –	0 points
Occasional or mild problems –	2 points
Frequent or severe problems –	4 points

9. Find it very difficult to lose weight, despite eating less or exercising more?

No –	0 points
Yes –	5 points

10. Suffer from swelling in the face?

No –   0 points
Occasional or mild problems –   2 points
Frequent or severe problems –   4 points

11. Find that your eyelids tend to be swollen and puffy?

No –   0 points
Occasional or mild problems –   2 points
Frequent or severe problems –   4 points

12. Find that you suffer from bags under your eyes?

No –   0 points
Occasional or mild problems –   2 points
Frequent or severe problems –   4 points

13. Feel that your memory is not what it used to be?

No –   0 points
Occasional or mild problems –   1 points
Frequent or severe problems –   2 points

14. Have yellowing of the skin, particularly in the palms of the hand and soles of the feet?

No –   0 points
Occasional or mild problems –   2 points
Frequent or severe problems –   4 points

15. Suffer from depression?

No –   0 points
Occasional or mild problems –   2 points
Frequent or severe problems –   4 points

16. Suffer from ankle swelling?

No –   0 points
Occasional or mild problems –   2 points
Frequent or severe problems –   4 points

17. Feel that your movements are somewhat slow?

No –   0 points
Occasional or mild problems –   3 points
Frequent or severe problems –   5 points

18. Suffer from a hoarse voice which is not connected to throat infection?

No –	0 points
Occasional or mild problems –	3 points
Frequent or severe problems –	5 points

19. Think that you are less mentally sharp than you used to be?

No –	0 points
Occasional or mild problems –	2 points
Frequent or severe problems –	4 points

20. Feel that your eyebrows are not as thick as they used to be?

No –	0 points
Yes –	5 points

Interpreting your score

0–9: low thyroid function is very unlikely

10–24: low thyroid function should be considered as a possibility and testing is recommended

25–39: low thyroid function is quite likely, testing is highly recommended

40 and above: low thyroid function is very likely, testing is highly recommended, and thyroid support is likely to be of benefit

Testing for low thyroid function

If answering the questionnaire above has aroused your suspicions about the efficiency of your thyroid gland, you may consider having your thyroid status assessed with a conventional blood test. My feeling is that while conventional blood testing may pick up some individuals with low thyroid function, it misses a lot of others. Let me explain why:

T4 and TSH – good in theory but not in practice

The conventional medical test for hypothyroidism involves drawing a blood sample and having this measured for TSH (thyroid stimulating hormone) and T4 (thyroxine). In theory, if thyroid function is low, then we should see this reflected in a low T4 level. As TSH tends to rise as T4 falls, the low T4 should also be accompanied by a high TSH level. Well, that's the theory, and some individuals with hypothyroidism do indeed have low T4 and high TSH levels. However, I have seen countless patients who appear to have significantly reduced thyroid function, and who respond to thyroid support, yet come up normal on the blood test. How is it that a sophisticated and expensive blood test could miss these individuals? Well, no one knows for certain, but there's a few good theories flying around.

1. The 'normal' ranges may not reflect what is truly normal

Once an individual's thyroid hormones have been measured, they are compared to levels believed to reflect what is normal. The normal ranges of thyroid hormones are determined by measuring the hormone levels of a group of people who are clinically deemed to have normal thyroid function (as assessed through their symptoms and signs). Assessing thyroid function clinically is notoriously difficult, and this certainly opens up the possibility that the population whose hormone levels were used to set the normal range actually included individuals with sub-optimal thyroid function. Bearing in mind the number of people who are passed off as normal but who respond well to thyroid treatment, this certainly does seem to be the case.

When hypothyroidism is suspected, doctors usually measure levels of TSH and T4. It is actually the level of TSH that is generally regarded as the best indicator of thyroid function. At the laboratory I normally use in London, there is more than a twenty-fold difference between the lowest and the highest 'normal' TSH levels. It does seem to me to be unlikely that such huge variation can be said to be representative of a truly normal population.

2. The body can become resistant to the effects of thyroid hormones

Having a hormone present in the blood is one thing, whether it's contributing much to the body's well-being is another. It is now well recognized, for instance, that individuals can become resistant to the hormone insulin, which may eventually lead to a problem with diabetes. It is possible, therefore, that individuals may have perfectly normal levels of thyroid hormones in their systems, but that their bodies are failing to respond.

3. Thyroid hormone levels may be altered by unrelated factors

Certain factors are known to artificially raise levels of T4 and reduce TSH levels. These factors include oestrogen hormones, such as those found in the oral contraceptive pill and hormone-replacement therapy, L-dopa (a medication used for Parkinson's disease), steroids and some forms of drugs used to treat psychiatric illness. If one or more of these factors is present in an individual, it might possibly corrupt the supposed accuracy of the blood test.

4. We're checking the wrong hormones

As we've discussed, the conventional tests for hypothyroidism involve checking T4 and TSH. Now, remember that it is in fact T3, not T4, that is the truly active form of the hormone. Why is it, then, that it is not routine to measure T3 levels in patients suspected of having, or being treated for, hypothyroidism? According to my local pathology laboratory, T3 levels are not checked because they are not considered 'cost-effective'. Read that as 'too expensive'. Whatever the reason for T3's omission in testing protocols, it does appear that in assessing and monitoring low thyroid function we may be failing to perform the most useful test of all.

Home testing of thyroid function

Earlier this century, an American doctor called Broda Barnes became very interested in the thyroid gland. After years of painstaking research, he came to the conclusion that conventional tests for thyroid function were inadequate. He discovered that it was possible to get a very good idea of thyroid function by measuring an individual's temperature first thing in the morning (1). The theory behind this is that in the absence of an infection, the body's temperature is essentially determined by thyroid function. Low thyroid function is therefore often reflected in a low body temperature.

To assess body temperature, Barnes developed the following test, which is usually referred to as the 'Barnes Test'.

> *Take a mercury thermometer and before you go to sleep shake it down and leave it by the bed. On waking and before getting up, place the bulb of the thermometer in your armpit and wait for a full ten minutes. Record the temperature.*

A mercury thermometer should be used, as these seem to be more accurate than the newer digital models currently available. The ten-minute cooking time is important because it is essential to make sure the mercury has risen to its maximum value before the reading is taken. Men and post-menopausal women can take their temperature on any day, as long as they don't have an infection. Because pre-menopausal women's temperatures tend to fluctuate with the hormonal cycle, Barnes suggested that the most accurate time to assess temperature was on the second, third or fourth day of the period.

The normal body temperature in the morning is between 36.6°C and 36.8°C (97.8°F and 98.2°F). A temperature of 36.4°C (97.4°F) or less strongly suggests a thyroid that is just not keeping pace.

Controversial but useful

Many doctors regard the Barnes Test to be too simple and homespun to be accurate. How could a self-administered, inexpensive test be better than the sophisticated, expensive laboratory tests we have come to rely upon? To be honest, I think this attitude to the Barnes Test stems from the fact that doctors are generally reliant on laboratory and other high-tech tests. While doctors are taught that treating the patient, rather than the test result, is a fundamental of good medical practice, I'm not sure this dictum is always adhered to. I clearly remember being told several times at medical school that any doctor should usually be able to make most diagnoses after taking a thorough history from the patient and then performing a clinical examination. The reality is that once doctors emerge from medical school, they find that the time they spend with their patients is very limited, and they are plainly unable to be as thorough as they would like. Many doctors therefore rely heavily on tests to reach a diagnosis, and this certainly seems to be true of thyroid disease.

I have lost count of the number of patients I have seen who have been signed off as having some mystery illness but who have many signs and symptoms of hypothyroidism. Yet, when the blood test comes back normal, they are told there is nothing wrong with them. Call me old-fashioned, but I still believe in the old ideals of listening to and observing patients. If, after seeing a patient, I suspect that they have low thyroid function, I get them to do the Barnes Test. If this comes up low, I will go on to discuss treatment options available to them, even if the blood test is normal.

What can cause low thyroid function?

A few theories have been put forward to explain the apparent prevalence of thyroid-related problems in the population. The front-runners are:

1. Iodine deficiency

Iodine is an essential nutrient for thyroid function. Without it, the thyroid gland tends to malfunction and enlarge, creating what is known as a goitre. Goitres, and other symptoms of hypothyroidism, are rare in Japan, a country with a population that has a very high intake of iodine. Iodine deficiency, and therefore goitres, is common in mountainous or inland areas that are far from the sea, such as the Alps and Pyrenees mountain areas in Europe, the Andes in South America and the Himalayas of Asia.

Another theory relating to iodine is that it may not do its job, even though it may be available in adequate amounts to the body. Iodine comes from a chemical group, which includes flourine, chlorine and bromine. These substances are becoming increasingly more common in the environment, and some scientists think that they may interfere with the way iodine is utilized by the body.

2. Chemical pollutants

There is some evidence that goitres can occur as a result of poisoning by chemical substances. The increasing prevalence of pollutants in the environment might therefore be a factor in problems with hypothyroidism.

3. Genetic factors

Hypothyroidism can lead to increased susceptibility to infection and reduced sexual functioning. Because of these factors, many sufferers of hypothyroidism have not had the opportunity to pass their genes on to future generations. With the advent of antibiotics and effective thyroid treatments, this has all changed, meaning that the genes which may increase the likelihood of thyroid disease are now likely to be much more prevalent.

Treating a sluggish thyroid

So, you've got the symptoms of hypothyroidism and your temperature came up cool.

What are the options? In my view, there are principally three therapeutic options for treating the thyroid:

1. **The natural approach – nutrients and herbs**
2. **The conventional approach – thyroxine**
3. **The combination approach – thyroid extracts**

1. The natural approach

There are several herbs and nutrients which may be of benefit in supporting thyroid function. These are the best of the bunch:

Iodine – this is an essential component of the thyroid hormones. Without it, the thyroid simply cannot make these hormones in sufficient quantity. Supplementing with iodine, for instance in the form of kelp or dulce, may therefore help to improve thyroid function.

Caution

Iodine is one of those nutrients for which too much can be a bad thing. High levels of iodine may in fact suppress thyroid function. Do not exceed 500 mcg per day, unless under the instruction of a doctor with an interest in this area.

Selenium – this mineral participates in the conversion of T4 into T3, and a deficiency of selenium may stall this process (2). Low selenium may reduce the effectiveness of the thyroid hormones. Other studies have also linked low levels of selenium with hypothyroidism.

Caution

Very high levels of selenium may actually lower levels of T3. It is important, therefore, not to exceed 300 mcg per day, unless under the advice of a doctor with an interest in the area.

Vitamin A – this has a very important role to play in thyroid function, and a deficiency of this nutrient does seem to significantly affect thyroid output.

Caution

Women who are pregnant or are planning pregnancy should not take more than 10,000 IU of vitamin A per day in supplement form.

Calcium and magnesium – important minerals which help in the regulation of the function of the thyroid and parathyroid glands.

L-Tyrosine – an amino acid that has an essential role to play in the formation of thyroid hormones. Tyrosine has also been found to help in the treatment of hypothyroidism.

L-Glutamine and L-Glycine – these two amino acids are required for normal functioning of the thyroid gland.

Specific supplements

Thyranol – a supplement that has been specifically formulated to support thyroid function. It's principle ingredients are dulce (a source of iodine), selenium, vitamin A, calcium, magnesium, tyrosine, glutamine and glycine. Thyranol also contains Siberian ginseng (which can help in the regulation of body temperature) and liquorice (which can give general support to the body's hormonal system). Long-term supplementation with Thyranol can help to stimulate thyroid function and reverse symptoms of hypothyroidism, including sensitivity to cold, fatigue and weight gain.

Contraindications

Thyranol should not be used during pregnancy or if pregnancy is being planned. Advice should always be sought from a doctor if conventional thyroid medication is being taken.

Availability

Details of how to obtain Thyranol can be found in the section entitled 'Useful Information' at the back of the book under the name *VitaTech*.

2. The conventional approach

The conventional medical approach to hypothyroidism is centred on the use of a synthetic version of the hormone thyroxine (T4). This is normally administered at a dose of 50–100 mcg per day, and increased in doses of 50 mcg every three or four weeks until blood results come into the normal range. The usual maintenance dose is between 100 and 200 mcg.

Certainly, some hypothyroid individuals feel significant benefit from taking thyroxine in the right dose. However, there are also many others who do not. Often, individuals who have been diagnosed as hypothyroid feel little or no better when receiving thyroxine treatment.

One reason for this may be that some individuals may have a problem converting thyroxine in to T3, the active form of the hormone. If you are currently taking thyroxine and feel it is not doing as much for you as you would like, it might be worth adding a selenium supplement to your regime, as this helps in the conversion of thyroxine to T3. Take 200 mcg per day.

In addition to thyroxine, the thyroid also secretes a hormone called di-iodotyrosine. Some doctors believe that this hormone has a more important effect than thyroxine in regulating thyroid gland function (4). This may help to explain why some individuals fail to feel real benefit from treatment with thyroxine alone.

3. The combination approach

Some doctors, usually naturally orientated ones, recommend supplements that contain actual thyroid tissue. These extracts, often referred to as thyroid glandulars, are usually made from cow or pig thyroid, and contain not just T4, but also T3. It is believed that the range of hormones available in a glandular supplement is much more likely to have a beneficial effect on hypothyroid individuals than the single hormone conventional treatment.

I have seen many patients who have not done well on thyroxine do much better once they have switched to a glandular supplement. Individuals who still feel cold, tired and are continuing to struggle with their weight on thyroxine, often perk up, warm up and start losing weight within a few weeks of switching therapies.

The most widely used thyroid glandular in the USA is a product called Armour desiccated thyroid. Often, patients are started on ¼–½ grain of this product per day, and the dose is then increased by ¼–½ grain increments every seven to ten days, until the patient feels well. Adults usually require a maintenance dose of between one and three grains a day.

Apart from containing a range of hormones (rather than just one), are there any other advantages for using a thyroid glandular over thyroxine? Individuals who start on thyroxine usually take it for the rest of their lives. This doesn't seem to be so true for those individuals on thyroid glandulars. It seems that after a period of treatment (between one and two years is typical) it is possible for individuals to wean themselves off thyroid glandulars without ill effect. Why this should be is not known for sure, but it is thought that glandular products may give the thyroid the opportunity to rest and recover in time. I have a strong suspicion that thyroid recovery of this nature is even more likely if other thyroid supportive measures are taken. I often find that the best results are achieved through using a combination of nutrients, herbs and glandular based products.

Caution

I strongly recommend that anyone considering using thyroid glandulars should work with a doctor with experience and expertise in this area. Thyroid glandulars must be used with special caution in individuals with a history of heart disease. Thyroid glandulars do have the potential to produce side effects such as anxiety, nervousness, palpitations, excessive weight loss and insomnia, if taken in excess.

Monitoring your progress

With the appropriate support, your thyroid function should improve in time. As it does, you may start to notice changes in your health such as improvements in your levels of energy, both physical and mental, and a lessened tendency towards depression, if this is a feature in you. Quite importantly, individuals who address an underlying thyroid problem almost invariably begin to lose weight, too. This is usually not dramatic, but it usually leads to very significant weight loss in the long term. In my view, the very best way to monitor the progress of your thyroid function is to do the Barnes Test from time to time. I have found in practice that symptoms of low thyroid do not resolve unless the temperature approaches normal, and that the temperature correlates very well with the overall functioning of the thyroid.

Case Study

Rosemary L is a 42-year-old company secretary

I only started having problems with weight once I hit my thirties. I had always managed to keep my weight down when I was younger without any problem. Most of the time, I didn't even think about what to eat, I just ate it! The problems started about 10 years ago. My weight started to creep up, despite the fact that nothing had changed. I started to have to be a little bit more careful about what I ate, but still my weight continued to rise. When I was 35 years old, I went to see my doctor. I asked him if it could be my thyroid. My mother has a thyroid problem and has been on tablets for over twenty years. Apart from the weight gain, I had really started to feel the cold, which I remember my mother used to suffer from terribly. My doctor agreed to run a test, which came back normal. Still the pounds piled on. By the time I was 40, I was more than 30 lbs overweight.

A friend of mine had been to see a naturopath who had helped her lose weight and regain her health by suggesting she took certain foods out of her diet. However, when I went to see him, he explained that food sensitivity was not my problem, but that I had symptoms of a sluggish thyroid. I did the temperature test for a few days and this averaged out at 96°F.

I started to take a nutritional supplement recommended by the naturopath designed to help stimulate the thyroid, along with a supplement of thyroid extract. It took me a while to find the right dose of the extract supplement, but after a few weeks I found I was starting to lose weight. I noticed a real lift in energy, felt much livelier in the morning and just had more oomph. Gradually, my sensitivity to cold went away. I eventually lost about 25 pounds over an eight-month period. I am thrilled about the weight loss, but I am also happy to have regained my health. Getting on top of my thyroid problem really did wake me up to how much my general health had slipped over the years.

Summary

● Undiagnosed low thyroid function plays a major role in many individuals' problems with excess weight.

● Other common symptoms of low thyroid function include sensitivity to cold, cold hands and feet, dry skin and hair, puffiness around the eyes, low mood and lethargy.

● The conventional blood tests designed to diagnose low thyroid function appear to miss a significant proportion of sufferers.

● Diagnosing hypothyroidism may be better done on the basis of an individual's symptoms and the Barnes temperature test.

● The treatment options for a sluggish thyroid include thyroxine (conventional treatment), herbs and nutrients, and thyroid glandulars.

● The Barnes Test is generally a good guide to how well the thyroid is responding to treatment.

● Supporting the thyroid with appropriate agents can lead to significant weight loss and a considerable improvement in general health.

CHAPTER 5

Eat Lean

It stands to reason that if there's one sure way to accumulate fat, it's to eat it. Now, while some fats (actually, *most* fats) in the diet are not good for your health, other fats (known as essential fatty acids) are positively beneficial. They play an important role in a range of processes, including skin health, hormonal balance, immune activity and mental function. In this chapter we'll be taking a close look at fat, discussing the health effects of the different types of fat and exploring ways of making healthier choices about types of fat.

The fats of life

Fats are basically made up of chains of carbon atoms to which hydrogen atoms are attached. There are two basic forms of fats: saturated fats and unsaturated fats. Saturated fats contain as many hydrogen atoms as is chemically possible, while unsaturated fats don't. Saturated fats are found in animal products such as pork, ham, bacon, beef, lamb, cold meats, sausage, hot dogs, butter, cream, yoghurt and cheese. The one significant non-animal source of saturated fat is coconut (palm) oil. It is thought that an excessive consumption of saturated fats predisposes to many health problems, including heart disease, stroke and some forms of cancer.

Unsaturated fats are found in margarine and vegetable oils such as sunflower, corn and safflower oils. For thirty years or more, unsaturated fats and oils have been touted as healthy alternatives to their saturated counterparts. However, there is growing evidence that the consumption of many unsaturated fats increases the risk of a range of medical conditions.

The unsaturated fats to avoid are those that are often described as 'partially hydrogenated'. These fats and oils are often made from a fairly decent vegetable oil, which has then been refined, heated and then exposed to hydrogen to change its properties as a foodstuff. While these processes may be good news for the food manufacturers, they are bad news for you. The body just isn't used to dealing with partially hydrogenated fats, which are essentially a recent food industry invention. As a result, partially hydrogenated fats reek havoc in the body and are increasingly linked to the development of a variety of conditions including arthritis, pre-menstrual syndrome, heart disease, cancer and increased susceptibility to infections.

Partially hydrogenated fats are found in abundance in margarine, but also appear in many processed foods including bread, crackers, biscuits, cakes, mayonnaise, salad cream and crisps and other deep-fried snacks. For the sake of your weight and of your health, these foods, in addition to those high in saturated fat, should be avoided wherever possible.

How much fat is in that food?

The standard Western diet is packed with fat. The health implications of this are enormous, and so cutting down on our intake of fat makes good sense for the majority of us. If we look at the nutritional information panel on the packaging of a food item, we can find out what percentage of the product contains fat. For instance, a 100 g (3.5 oz) serving of cream cheese contains 30 g (1 oz) of fat, meaning that 30% of the product is fat. This is useful information but, from a nutritional point of view, what we really need to know is not so much its fat percentage, but the percentage of calories contributed by the fat. As a general guide, we should aim to ensure that no more than 30% of the total calories we eat come from fat. So, as long as we choose foods for which this is the case, then our diet is bound to be relatively healthy as far as fat is concerned.

Calculating the percentage of calories contributed by fat

Each gram of fat contains nine calories of energy. So, to calculate the total number of fat calories in a product, we have to take the total number of grams of fat it contains and multiply this by nine. To get the percentage of calories contributed by fat, we have to divide this figure by the total number of calories in the product, and then multiply by a hundred.

For example, let's say your favourite supermarket pre-prepared chicken dish contains 5g of fat and a total of 250 calories. The percentage of calories contributed by fat would be:

$$\frac{5 \text{ (number of grams of fat)} \times 9}{\text{Total number of calories: 250}} \times 100 = 18\%$$

If the nutritional value of a food is expressed per unit weight, say per 100 g, then the figures are different, but the result is the same. In this case, the percentage of calories contributed by fat would be:

$$\frac{2.5 \text{ (number of grams of fat per 100 g)} \times 9}{\text{Total number of calories per 100 g:}} \times 100 = 18\%$$

You can make your own calculations for your favourite foods. However, just to make things a little easier for you, here is a list of some commonly eaten foods and how they fare in the fat stakes:

Percentage of calories contributed by fat

75% or more
bacon
beef – most cuts and hamburgers
coleslaw
cream – all forms
cream cheese
frankfurters and hot dogs
ham – untrimmed
nuts (walnuts, peanuts, brazils etc)
peanut butter
pork – including sausage, ribs
   and loin

50%–75%
cheese (blue, cheddar etc)
chicken – roasted with skin
chocolate
eggs
ice cream (full–fat)
pork – trimmed ham and loin
   lamb (chops and rib)
tuna in oil (not drained)

40%–50%
beef – lean T-bone and lean
   hamburger
chicken (fried)
ice cream (regular)
mackerel
milk, full-fat
salmon (canned)
sardines
yoghurt, full-fat

30%–40%
chicken – roasted without skin
milk, semi-skimmed
pizza
seafood

tuna in oil (drained)
turkey – roast, dark meat
yoghurt – low-fat
white fish – halibut, haddock

20% – 30%
beef – lean sirloin
cod
liver
oysters
soups – tomato and vegetable

less than 20%
beans, pulses and lentils
bread
breakfast cereals
cottage cheese
frozen yoghurt
fruits
tuna in brine
turkey – roasted white meat
vegetables

(adapted from Jane Brody's Nutrition Book (New York: Norton 1981)

Now, if we're aiming to keep our percentage of calories contributed by fat to below the 30% mark, then this means eating a diet rich in fruits, vegetables, beans, pulses, lean meat and fish. For more information about how to make healthy food choices and how best to prepare the food you choose to eat, read on.

Fish first

I know it won't come as an amazing revelation to you that the healthiest option here is fish. Oily fish, such as mackerel, salmon and trout, contain fats that have an important role to play in health, particularly in the prevention of heart disease (more about these healthy fats later). Avoid fish which has been battered or covered in breadcrumbs, as this is likely to contain more unhealthy fat than its fresh variety.

Poultry is relatively low in fat, as long as the skin is discarded before cooking. If you do buy red meat, opt for lean cuts which have had the fat already trimmed.

Choosing dairy products

Skimmed milk is the healthiest form of milk because it contains virtually no fat. Even semi-skimmed milk makes a healthy alternative to full-fat milk as it has approximately half the fat content (and about 30% of calories contributed by fat).

Cheeses basically come in ripened (e.g. cheddar, Swiss, brie and parmesan) and unripened (e.g. cottage, cream, mozzarella, ricotta) forms. The unripened cheeses generally contain less fat and cholesterol compared with the ripened cheeses and are therefore preferred. However, even the unripened cheeses are pretty fatty and should be kept to a minimum in the diet. An exception here is cottage cheese, which has less than 20% of its calories contributed by fat.

Live natural unsweetened yoghurt is the healthiest form of yoghurt. Fruit yoghurts tend to contain large amounts of sugar or artificial sweeteners such as aspartame. Fresh fruit added to natural yoghurt is a great combination.

Preparing foods

Apart from making low-fat food choices, the other major area in which we can reduce fat intake is in food preparation. This section looks at how food may be prepared and cooked with a view to reducing fat consumption.

Avoid shallow- and deep-fried food

These methods of cooking add significant quantities of fat to food and are therefore best avoided. In addition, heating oil to a high temperature can change the nature of the oil, making it potentially harmful to the body.

Low-fat cooking

Many cooking methods do not require the addition of fat to enhance the cooking process. Probably the most healthy of all cooking methods is steaming. Steaming is fast, fat-free and causes minimal nutrient loss. This method of cooking is suitable for fish and vegetables.

Boiling is an alternative to steaming but the nutrient losses tend to be greater with this method of cooking. Somewhere in between boiling and steaming is poaching, which is most often used to cook fish.

Roasting is a relatively low-fat method of cooking joints of meat and poultry. No oil or fat should be added before or during the cooking process. The meat should be put on a rack so that the fat has the opportunity to drain away from the meat while it is cooking.

Grilling is a low-fat method of cooking and is suitable for cooking thinner cuts of meat, poultry cuts, fish and certain vegetables such as tomatoes and peppers. Char-grilled food should be avoided, as there is some association between this method of cooking and the risk of certain cancers.

Use non-stick kitchen utensils

Should you have to fry food, then using a non-stick frying pan or saucepan can cut down on the amount of oil or fat needed.

Cut back the fat

Removing as much fat as possible prior to cooking meals such as casseroles and stews will help to ensure that as little fat as possible ends up on the plate. Also, after cooking, chill meats, stews and soups so that the fat rises to the top and solidifies. This can then be removed and discarded before re-heating and serving.

Use low-fat dairy products in recipes

Full-fat milk can be replaced with skimmed or semi-skimmed versions. Cream can be mixed half-and-half with low-fat natural yoghurt or fromage frais. Use the low-fat version of cheese if this is required in a recipe.

Cut down on the amount of fat you add during cooking

Even when some form of fat, such as butter, is called for in a recipe, the quantity of fat can usually be reduced by a third without affecting texture or taste.

Low-fat fallacy

Bearing in mind the mania regarding fat consumption that has gripped the nation, it's hardly surprising that low-fat foods are becoming increasingly more profitable for the food manufacturing companies. Supermarket shelves are full of products declaring themselves to be 'low in fat', 'lite', or 'cholesterol-free'. The question is, are they really any healthier than their full-fat versions, or is their healthy image just a load of marketing hype? Using the percentage of calories contributed by fat calculation, we can see just how well (or not) these claims hold up.

Using cream cheese as an example, we find that the 30% fat in the full-fat variety converts to 86% of its calories coming from fat. So, cream cheese has no problems making it into the unhealthy bin. However, is its low-fat version any better? At just 15% fat, it certainly looks as if it might be. However, doing the sums reveals that the percentage of calories coming from fat is still a whopping 73. This hardly classifies it as a health food.

Another problem with many low-fat foods is that they often contain spoonfuls of sugar. Products such as low-fat ice cream, biscuits and cakes may have less fat than their original versions, but they're usually full to the brim with sugar. As sugar has health hazards of its own, it is unlikely to help you shed your surplus pounds (for more information about the effect of sugar on weight and health read chapter 3, *Balance Your Blood Sugar*).

Good fats

In our food supply fats exist that have important roles to play in the maintenance of weight and health. These fats are commonly referred to as the essential fatty acids (EFAs). EFAs come in two main forms, known as the omega-3 and omega-6 fatty acids. Omega-6 fatty acids are present in all the common oils found in the human diet, including sunflower oil, safflower oil, corn oil, sesame oil and rape seed oil. Omega-3 fatty acids can be found in linseed (flaxseed) oil and oily fish such as salmon, trout and mackerel. Omega-3 and omega-6 fatty acids have quite distinct, yet complementary, roles and contribute to many bodily processes, including hormone balance, skin health, immune-system function and the regulation of cholesterol levels in the blood. Together, omega-3 and omega-6 fatty acids are thought to be effective in combating conditions as diverse as heart disease, cancer, arthritis, allergies and pre-menstrual syndrome.

Using healthy fats to get back in balance

In the Western world we tend to get plenty of omega-6 fatty acids through our diets, but the amount of omega-3 we consume is small by comparison. Many of us therefore suffer from a deficiency of omega-3 fatty acids, manifestations of which include dry skin, water retention, high blood pressure and an increased susceptibility to infection. The relative lack of omega-3 in the diet has led to the increasing popularity of linseed oil, which contains omega-3 and omega-6 fats in a ratio of 3:1. Many nutritionists recommend linseed oil because of its high omega-3 content. While linseed oil may be useful in overcoming omega-3 deficiency, it may not be the best oil for continued use. The most up-to-date research suggests that, in the long term, we should consume three times as much omega-6 fat as omega-3.

Hemp-seed oil contains the essential fats in precisely this ratio. Also, unlike other common seed oils, hemp-seed oil contains a type of fat called gamma-linolenic acid (the active ingredient in evening primrose oil), which has specific health-giving properties. Because of the blend of essential fats it contains, hemp seed oil has come to be recognized as nature's most perfectly balanced oil for long-term use (1).

Hemp-seed oil does not contain the mind-altering substances normally associated with the hemp plant. The oil looks similar to a dark olive oil but has a flavour similar to sunflower oil. It can be taken straight off the spoon, used as a condiment for food or as an ingredient for a healthy salad dressing. The oil should not be heated, as this affects the chemical nature of the oil dramatically, reducing its beneficial effects in the body. Details of how hemp-seed oil can be obtained by mail order can be found in the 'Useful Information' section at the back of the book under the name *Advanced Herbals*.

Eat fat and lose weight

New research is emerging that suggests that a certain type of fat, known as conjugated linoleic acid (CLA), can actually help speed up weight loss. CLA appears to help the body regulate fat and protein. Specifically, it appears to assist the body in burning fat and making protein (muscle) (2). And where can CLA be found in the diet? Red meat and dairy products. But, before you start to gorge yourself on steak and cheese, remember that these foods are not recommended in quantity because of their high content of unhealthy saturated fat. The downside of saturated fats does appear to outweigh the beneficial effects of CLA. Another way round this problem is to take supplements of CLA, which are becoming increasingly available. The recommended dose is 1,200 mg three times a day before meals.

Fat-friendly menus

Breakfast

1. Low-sugar or no-sugar breakfast cereal based on oats, wheat, corn or rice, with skimmed milk, fruit and seeds (sesame, sunflower or pumpkin).

2. Wholegrain rye or wheat-based bread or toast with 'no sugar added' jam.

3. Fresh fruit salad with low-fat natural yoghurt.

4. Blended fruit smoothie made with strawberries, low-fat yoghurt, ice and a small amount of honey.

5. Grilled kippers and tomatoes with wholegrain toast.

Lunches

1. Fresh vegetable soup and rye crackers.

2. Skinless chicken salad sandwich on wholegrain rye or wheat bread.

3. Skinless chicken or tuna salad dressed with extra virgin olive oil and lemon juice.

Suppers

1. Grilled or poached trout or salmon with steamed vegetables.

2. Fish pie casserole with baked potato and steamed vegetables.

3. Pasta with tomato-based sauce and salad dressed with extra virgin olive oil and sesame seeds.

Case Study

Roger J is a 54-year-old management consultant

My work takes me all over the world. On a long project I might be based for months in a foreign country, spending the week there and flying home at the weekend. At other times I can go through spells of getting on and off planes, country hopping and living out of a suitcase. What this means is that most of my meals are eaten in restaurants, hotels and on planes. In the past, it would be one rich meal after the other.

Over the years, I got bigger and bigger. I was 12 stones when I was at college, but ended up at 15½ stones by the time I was 50. I just tried to ignore the fact that I was putting on increasing amounts of weight. Every time I had a company medical they would tell me that I needed to lose weight, but with my lifestyle I just couldn't see how. Then, two years ago, a medical showed up a high cholesterol level. This triggered me into action.

I became very aware of the amount of fat that I was eating. I started to look carefully at menus and made a conscious effort to make healthier choices. My tactics were simple: if I was eating a restaurant meal, I would always have either a clear soup or salad as a starter. For the main course I would eat fish, often salmon or sea bass, grilled or poached, with plenty of vegetables. I read that extra virgin olive oil was good news, so I ordered this and put it on my salad and dipped my bread in it, too. Sometimes I would eat meat, but not often. Cheese got the heave-ho. I pre-ordered the low-fat option when booking flights. If I was away from home, I started to have fruit or fruit salad for breakfast. Occasionally, if I was hungry, I might order some fish or poached eggs on toast, maybe with some mushrooms and tomatoes.

I'm not in the habit of weighing myself, but I certainly noticed that after only a month or so of eating to this pattern I was lighter. Suit trousers that were just a bit too tight were feeling comfortable again. I was much less sluggish after meals, and somehow less bloated, too. Four months after I started my low-fat regime, the company doctor checked my cholesterol and it was better, only slightly above normal. My weight continued to decline, and over the course of eight or nine months I lost a stone and a half. The following year I lost about another stone. I weigh under 13 stones now, perhaps 10 or 12 pounds heavier than I was thirty years ago but I'm happy with that, and I haven't had to turn my life upside down to get here.

Summary

- The diet should be based around foods which have no more than 30% of the calories contributed by fat.

- Foods such as fruits, vegetables, beans, pulses, lean meat and fish should form the basis of the diet.

- The diet should be rich in foods high in essential fatty acids, including oily fish, extra virgin olive oil and raw nuts and seeds.

- For all-round health benefit, hemp-seed oil is the best balanced oil for long-term use.

- Limiting your intake of saturated and other unhealthy fats makes good sense for weight control and general health.

6

Eliminate Your Allergies

Foods such as wholemeal bread and skimmed milk are generally regarded as ideal components of a healthy, weight-reducing diet. Adhering to the commonly lauded 'high-fibre, low fat' ideal, these foods feature heavily in many weight-loss regimes. Despite their healthy image, it appears that these, and some other foods which are generally regarded as 'healthy', may be at the root of many people's weight problems. Scientific evidence is amassing to suggest that excess weight – and a whole host of other health problems – may be related to unwanted reactions to everyday foods.

In this chapter we shall be exploring this concept, which is often referred to as 'food allergy' or 'food intolerance'. In general terms, this idea has not gained wide acceptance by the conventional medical establishment. Most doctors and dieticians believe that food reactions are rare and only affect a small proportion of the population. However, in recent years there has been growing interest and research into a type of food reaction that cannot be identified by conventional testing, but which is nonetheless common, and quite often a factor in excess weight and a variety of medical conditions. For many individuals, identifying the foods to which they are sensitive is a critical step towards bringing about lasting and healthy weight loss.

Understanding food reactions

To understand how food reactions occur, we need first to gain an understanding of the concepts of food digestion and absorption.

Digestion

Digestion takes place in the digestive tract. This begins at the mouth and runs right down to the anus *(see below)*. The parts of the digestive tract actively involved in the process of digestion are the mouth, stomach and small intestine.

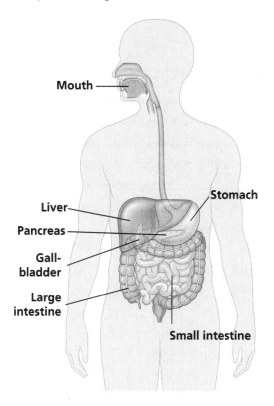

Mouth — Liver — Pancreas — Gall-bladder — Large intestine — Stomach — Small intestine

The mouth

Digestion of food starts in the mouth. The very act of chewing stimulates the secretion of digestive juices lower down in the gut. Chewing also mixes food with an enzyme to start the digestion of starchy foods such as bread, potatoes, rice and pasta. By breaking food up, chewing also increases the surface area available for contact with the digestive juices, allowing them to penetrate the food and do their digestive work.

The stomach

The stomach secretes acid to start the digestion of protein-based foods such as meat, fish and dairy products.

The small intestine

Once food leaves the stomach, it passes into the small intestine. Here it is subjected to the action of digestive enzymes to continue the digestive process. Some of these are found in the wall of the gut itself, while some of these are secreted by a gland called the pancreas. Bile, secreted by the gallbladder, also works on the food and helps with the digestion of fat.

The purpose of digestion is to break food up into pieces small enough to be absorbed through the gut wall and into the bloodstream. The main constituents in the diet that need to be broken down in this way are fats, starches and proteins. Fats themselves are made up of chains of smaller molecules known as fatty acids.

Starches are actually composed of chains of sugar molecules, while proteins are comprised of molecules called amino acids.

The total surface area of the small intestine is about the size of a tennis court. It is composed of finger-like structures called villi. Each villus is covered in much smaller structures called microvilli. The presence of villi and microvilli increases the surface area of the gut available for absorption.

Digestion and food sensitivity

Conventional medical wisdom dictates that before food is absorbed through the gut wall into the bloodstream, it is first broken down into its smallest molecular constituents. In other words, fats are broken down into fatty acids, starches are broken down into individual sugar molecules and proteins are broken down into amino acids. If this was the case, then the reality would be that there is very limited potential for foods to cause adverse reactions in the body. The basic molecular constituents of food would be too small to be seen as foreign by the body.

A new way of looking at food sensitivity

In recent years, however, this conventional view of digestion and food sensitivity has been challenged. There is emerging evidence to suggest that it is possible for food to pass into the bloodstream in a partially digested form. When this happens, there is enormous potential for unwanted reactions to food in the body.

Adverse food reactions can occur when partially digested food is absorbed into the bloodstream and comes into contact with the immune system. The immune system is made up of various types of white blood cells. The function of these cells is to protect the body from anything that may be perceived as foreign, and therefore a threat, to the body. The immune cells are constantly in 'search and destroy' mode, continually on the lookout for harmful organisms such as bacteria and viruses.

However, undigested or partially digested food may also trigger the immune defences, and this may lead to a wide variety of conditions. The immune reactions caused by food can occur anywhere, which opens up a host of possibilities for any manner of conditions or symptoms. Conditions believed to have no specific underlying cause, such as irritable bowel syndrome and eczema, are, in fact, often due to the body's reactions to food. In Britain, these unwanted food reactions are often termed 'food intolerance'. In the USA, the more commonly used term is 'food allergy'. To avoid confusion, the rest of the chapter will refer to these adverse food reactions as 'food sensitivity'.

The immune system and food sensitivity

The white cells of the immune system contain a sub-class of cells known as the lymphocytes. A particular type of lymphocyte, the B-lymphocyte, is responsible for making substances called antibodies (also known as immunoglobulins). The antibodies produced by the B-lymphocytes help the body neutralize or destroy any invading organisms. There are five different forms of antibodies, two of which, IgE and IgM (the prefix Ig stands for 'immunoglobulin'), are of importance to us with regard to food sensitivity.

IgE sensitivity

IgE can bind to immune cells called mast cells, triggering the release of a substance called histamine. This is the substance that causes the sneezing and runny eyes characteristic of hay fever. In hay fever, the IgE production and histamine release occurs as a response to pollen, although sometimes these reactions can be triggered by food. If an individual eats a strawberry and quickly develops a red rash, this is almost definitely an IgE reaction. Some childhood food sensitivities are IgE related. This type of food reaction is well accepted by the conventional medical establishment but plays little, if any, role in the processes that may ultimately lead to weight gain and chronic health problems.

IgG sensitivity

The sort of reactions that may contribute to weight gain can often be related to the production of IgG. If blood samples are drawn from food-sensitive individuals, it is often possible to detect IgG antibodies to specific foods. There is a theory that the IgG antibodies produced in response to certain foods can also cause the immune response to spill over into the body's own tissues, and it is this process that is often at the root of many health conditions.

IgG food reactions tend to come on much more slowly than IgE reactions. While IgE reactions are pretty much immediate, IgG reactions can take two or more days to show themselves. Also, while the symptoms of IgE sensitivity tend to be quite obvious (vomiting, rash, etc), those related to IgG tend to be subtler. It is not uncommon for IgG reactions to produce vague symptoms, including fatigue or general feelings of malaise.

However, it is not true to say that food sensitivity is at the root of all cases of these symptoms and conditions. Many of these conditions have several potential underlying mechanisms. Nevertheless, if an individual is suffering from one or more of these problems, it is often useful to consider food sensitivity as a potential trigger factor. What is more, it is quite common for an individual to exhibit several seemingly unconnected symptoms at the same time but which turn out to have the same underlying cause.

Some of the symptoms and conditions thought to be related to IgG-mediated food sensitivity include:

Headache

Migraine

Fatigue

Fluid retention

Muscle aches and fibromyalgia

Stomach and duodenal ulcers

Depression

Anxiety

Hyperactivity in children

Poor mental concentration/ brain fog

Excessive production of mucus/catarrh

Attacks of gallbladder inflammation (cholecystitis)

Diarrhoea

Constipation

Abdominal bloating

Irritable bowel syndrome

Crohn's disease

Eczema

Rheumatoid arthritis

Weight gain

Is food intolerance your problem?

The following questionnaire is designed to help you ascertain whether food sensitivity is a problem for you. Score each question as indicated, and then add up your total score.

1. Do you feel lethargic soon after eating?
No –   0 points
Occasional or mild problems –   2 points
Frequent or severe problems –   4 points

2. Do you often feel better if you don't eat?
No –   0 points
Marginally better –   2 points
Much better –   4 points

3. Did you have problems such as colic, glue ear, ear infections, eczema, asthma or recurrent tonsillitis as a child?
No –   0 points
Yes, occasional problems –   3 points
Yes, frequent and/or severe problems – 5 points

4. Do you have recurrent, unexplained symptoms?
No –   0 points
Occasional or mild problems –   2 points
Frequent or severe problems –   4 points

5. Do you suffer from excess mucus or catarrh formation in the throat, nose or sinuses?
No –   0 points
Occasional or mild problems –   2 points
Frequent or severe problems –   4 points

6. Do you feel particularly drawn to certain foods such as bread or cheese?
No –   0 points
Occasionally –   2 points
Frequently –   4 points

7. Do you have dark circles under your eyes?
No –   0 points
Yes –   2 points
Frequent or severe problems –   4 points

8. Do you suffer from fluid retention? (Tight rings, puffy face or ankles and a weight which fluctuates by two or more pounds from day to day are classic signs.)

No –   0 points
Occasional or mild problems –   2 points
Frequent or severe problems –   4 points

9. Do you suffer from irritable bowel syndrome?

No –   0 points
Occasional or mild problems –   1 points
Frequent or severe problems –   2 points

10. Do you suffer from eczema, hives (urticaria) or undiagnosed rash?

No –   0 points
Occasional or mild problems –   2 points
Frequent or severe problems –   4 points

Interpreting your score

0–9:   food sensitivity is unlikely
10–20:   food sensitivity should be considered as a possibility and testing (see below) is recommended
21 and above: food sensitivity is very likely and testing is highly recommended

What causes food intolerance?

Many food intolerances start very early in life. There is even some evidence that children can become sensitized to food while they are still in the womb. Quite often foods are introduced into a child's diet when the intestinal tract and immune system are relatively immature. As a result, the child is unable to deal appropriately with that food, causing him or her to become sensitive to it. For example, infants who are bottle-fed often become sensitive to cow's milk formula feeds. This can manifest in a number of ways, but colic and eczema are common signs.

There is a theory that food intolerances are becoming more common because we are eating more and more foods that are relatively recent additions to our diet. It may be that we just have not had long enough to adjust to these new foods. For example, although we have cultivated and eaten wheat for many thousands of years, the form of wheat we eat now is quite different from the form of wheat we evolved on. Milk is another example. Although we have drunk milk for quite some time during our evolution, for many populations it was predominantly goat's and sheep's milk, not cow's milk, that they became accustomed to drinking. Pasteurization is also thought to be an important factor in the seemingly increasing prevalence of cow's milk sensitivity.

Poor digestion and food sensitivity

It is highly possible that inadequate digestion of food is a feature in food sensitivity. The less well food is digested, the more likely it is to leak into the bloodstream in a partially digested form. Poor digestion may be related to a range of factors, including inadequate chewing, lack of stomach acid or insufficient pancreatic digestive enzymes (see page 121).

Leakiness in the gut and food sensitivity

The lining of the gut wall performs many functions, one of which is to ensure that food is not absorbed until it has been properly digested. However, in certain circumstances, the gut wall may become 'leaky', allowing larger molecules than is desirable into the bloodstream (see page 121).

Food sensitivity and weight gain

Now we have some idea of how food sensitivity comes about, but how does this relate to weight gain? There is a wealth of anecdotal evidence to suggest that food sensitivity is a common factor in weight gain. These findings are supported scientifically, too (1). The precise mechanism for the role of food sensitivity in excess weight is unknown, but the most likely explanations, however, are:

1. Food sensitivity causes fluid retention

Fluid retention is a common symptom of food sensitivity, especially in women. Common manifestations of this include swelling of the face (especially in the morning), swelling of the ankles (especially at the end of the day), weight fluctuation of a few pounds from day to day, weight gain of a few pounds in the few days prior to a period and finger swelling, often causing rings on the fingers to feel uncomfortably tight.

The likely cause of these symptoms is that food reactions are causing inflammation in the body's smallest blood vessels (the capillaries), causing them to leak. Fluid, which is normally kept within the vessel, can then escape into the tissues, leading to waterlogging. While fluid retention is likely to be a factor in many cases of weight gain, it is unlikely to be the sole cause in most people. Many individuals find that attending to their food sensitivities brings about losses in weight that are too great to be explained by this phenomenon alone.

2. Food sensitivity jams the metabolism

To generate energy from food, it needs to be in its completely digested form. The food that makes it through into the system in a partially digested form cannot be used to generate energy. Worse than this, it is possible that partially digested food may interfere with the normal food-burning reactions in the body. You can imagine large food molecules gumming up the works, preventing the efficient burning of properly digested food. If this is true, then the body is going to have difficulty burning food to make energy, perhaps explaining why most food-sensitive individuals cite weight gain and fatigue as two of their major symptoms.

3. Food sensitivity lowers thyroid function

In medicine, some conditions are described as 'auto-immune' diseases. In these conditions, the body's immune system seems to react against its own tissues, leading to problems in the parts of the body where reactions take place. Examples of auto-immune conditions include rheumatoid arthritis, where there is a reaction against the tissues that line certain joints, and childhood diabetes, where immune reactions destroy the cells in the pancreas that make insulin. Another site of the body which may be susceptible to auto-immune reactions is the thyroid. The thyroid is the gland chiefly responsible for regulating the metabolism (see chapter 4, *Keep Up the Heat*). If the thyroid function declines for any reason, weight generally goes up. Low thyroid function is an under-recognized cause of weight gain.

Testing for food sensitivity

If you think that you have food intolerance, there are a number of methods that can be used to ascertain which foods are causing the problem. These include:

Scratch testing and IgE blood testing

The scratch test, also known as the prick test or patch test, involves breaching the outer layer of the skin and introducing a tiny amount of the food or other substance (e.g. animal hair, pollen, etc) to be tested. Redness and swelling at the site of the test indicates a sensitivity to whatever is being tested. Blood tests also exist which detect IgE antibodies to specific foods. Because IgE reactions almost certainly have no bearing on weight, these tests have no relevance here.

Cytotoxic testing

This test is performed by mixing immune cells with various food extracts and then ascertaining which foods caused reactions in the immune cells. This test is usually interpreted by a technician, who uses a microscope to assess whether the immune cells have reacted and to what degree. In this sense, the test is subject to human interpretation and the possibility of error, though an experienced technician is likely to give an accurate interpretation of the results.

The ALCAT test

ALCAT stands for the Antigen Leucocyte Cellular Antibody Test. It is quite similar to the cytotoxic test, except that the white cells' reactions to foodstuffs are measured by a sophisticated piece of laboratory equipment, rather than a technician. It is possible that ALCAT is more accurate than cytotoxic testing, but this has not been proven and ALCAT is usually more expensive.

IgG testing

It is possible to detect IgG antibodies to specific foods using sophisticated biochemical techniques. There are two basic techniques which are used, the RAST (radioallergosorbent test) and ELISA (enzyme-linked immunoserological assay). These tests are thought to be quite reliable indicators of food sensitivity. It is believed that ELISA is more sensitive than RAST – and it is cheaper, too.

Electro-dermal testing

Practitioners of Chinese medicine believe that energy flows through various invisible tracts in the body, known as meridians. In the 1950s, a German doctor by the name of Reinholdt Voll discovered that you could derive much information about the health status of the body by measuring the electrical current flowing through the acupuncture points. Electro-dermal testing involves measuring the electrical current that flows through an acupuncture point, and then detecting any changes in this when the body is challenged with individual foods. In this form of testing, food extracts are put in the same circuit as the subject being tested. If adding the food changes the electrical current flow through the acupuncture point, then this suggests that there is a problem with the food. Some more sophisticated devices have foods stored on a computer in the form of the electromagnetic 'fingerprint' of that food.

In skilled hands, this method seems to give good results, which are instantaneous. Electro-dermal testing is relatively cheap compared to the blood tests that are available for diagnosing food sensitivity. Because it is economical and instantaneous, I have to say that I like this form of testing, but you should find a practitioner who has had plenty of testing experience.

Applied kinesiology

This is similar to electro-dermal testing except that the practitioner measures muscle strength in response to foods, rather than the electrical current flowing through the body. Typically, muscle strength is first ascertained by the practitioner pressing down on the subject's outstretched arm. This is repeated while challenging the subject with a range of suspect or common foods, either by having them hold them close to their body or by putting samples of food under the tongue. As with electro-dermal testing, the results are thought to be relatively accurate in skilled hands and they are instantaneous. Again, testing tends to be inexpensive when compared to blood tests to determine food intolerance.

The elimination diet

Many practitioners of nutritional medicine regard the elimination diet as the most accurate way of testing for food sensitivity. The concept is simple: all likely problem foods are removed from the diet for a period of time. Once the symptoms or condition(s) being treated alleviate, foods are added back into the diet, one at a time, and a note is made of which foods cause a recurrence of the symptoms.

Knowing which foods to eliminate from the diet is an art in itself. To help you, here is some guidance:

1. Eliminate all sources of wheat (a very common problem food) from the diet. This includes most breads, pasta, pastry, pizza, biscuits, cakes, wheat-based breakfast cereals, wheat crackers, breaded food, battered food and anything containing flour.

2. Eliminate milk, cheese and yoghurt from the diet (very common source of problems, especially milk and cheese).

3. Eliminate foods and drinks that you consume repeatedly, say on four or more days each week (the more of a food you eat, the more likely it is to be a problem).

4. Eliminate the foods and drinks you crave and think you might not be able to do without. These foods may have a stimulant or pick-me-up effect in you.

5. Eliminate the foods and drinks you suspect make you feel bad.

All these foods should be eliminated for two weeks.

Taking a food out of the diet is one thing, finding something to replace it with is another. The following table includes a list of the most common food sensitivities, with some viable alternatives.

Food Sensitivities and Alternatives

Problem foodstuff	**Alternative**
Wheat-based bread	100% Rye bread
	Rye crackers
	Rye pumpernickel bread
	Rice cakes
	Oat cakes

Problem foodstuff	Alternative
Wheat-based breakfast cereals	Oat muesli Porridge (oatmeal) Cornflakes Puffed rice Multi-grain cereals based on non-wheat grains such as amaranth, millet and rice
Pasta (durum wheat)	Vegetable, rice and corn-based pasta
Egg noodles	Rice noodles
Gluten-containing food (Wheat, oats, rye and barley)	Rice cakes Multi-grain cereals based on non-wheat grains such as amaranth, millet and rice. Rice Rice noodles Potato Polenta (corn meal)
Cow's milk	Sheep's milk Goat's milk Soya milk Rice milk
Cow's cheese	Goat's cheese Sheep's cheese (e.g. feta)
Cow's yoghurt	Sheep's yoghurt Goat's yoghurt Soya yoghurt
Coffee and tea	Herb and fruit teas Dandelion coffee Chicory/barley-based coffee substitutes

Generally speaking, the sort of meals most food-intolerant individuals find work for them are based on the following theme:

> Meat, fish, eggs (e.g. omelette or hard-boiled eggs) or tofu
> Vegetables
> Rice or potato

> For example:
> Roast chicken with steamed broccoli and carrots and roast potatoes
> Tuna salad with new potatoes
> Grilled salmon with salad and rice
> Omelette and salad
> Tofu casserole with rice and salad

If you do suffer from food sensitivity, you may well be feeling much better after a week or two on this regime. Many individuals whose excess weight is linked to food sensitivity find that they experience a sudden and dramatic fall in weight. It is not uncommon for individuals to lose four or five kilograms (ten or more pounds) in just a couple of weeks. Other commonly experienced improvements include increased energy, enhanced mental clarity and less problematic digestive function.

Elimination diet caution

It is worth noting that in the initial phase of an elimination diet, it is not uncommon for sensitive individuals to experience withdrawal reactions. A gnawing hunger, nasal stuffiness, inability to concentrate, fatigue, insomnia and nervousness are not uncommon symptoms. These reactions normally last for a few days, and very rarely longer than a week. The symptoms can be lessened by taking 1 gram of vitamin C every couple of hours or so.

Re-testing foods

If you are feeling better after a couple of weeks on the elimination diet, it's time to start testing foods. Take one of the foods you have eliminated and have a substantial portion of it one morning. A glass of milk at breakfast is an example. Over the next few hours you will need to look out for any symptoms which suggest food sensitivity. These include headache, itching, depression, fatigue, irritability and foggy thinking. If you get any reaction, make a note that the provoking food is one of your sensitivities and eliminate it again from your diet. If you have no reaction to your first exposure to the food, try it again at lunch and dinner. If by the following morning you are totally free from symptoms, provisionally add it to your safe list of foods.

For the next three days re-eliminate the food and keep a watchful eye out for any symptoms that suggest a food reaction. It is possible that the symptoms of a reaction can come on two or three days after a food or drink is consumed. If such a reaction occurs, you should suspect this food. If you still feel well after the three-day break, you can be pretty sure the foodstuff you are testing is fine for you.

In this way, proceed through the major foods you have eliminated, making a note of safe and unsafe foods as you go.

What if the elimination diet doesn't help?

If the elimination diet outlined above doesn't help you, there are two main possible explanations:

1. The foods to which you are sensitive were not eliminated from the diet.
2. That you don't have a food sensitivity problem.

To find out which of these is the case, it might be worthwhile eliminating more foods than the ones outlined on pages 95–97. A useful diet that you can try is what is known as the 'Stone Age' or 'Caveman Diet'.

The Stone Age diet

In this diet, all foods introduced after the advent of farming and animal domestication are eliminated from the diet. This means no grains (wheat, oats, rye, barley, rice and corn), dairy products (butter, milk, cheese, yoghurt, margarine), refined sugar, alcohol and food additives (including sweeteners). Eggs are often permitted on such a diet, but I prefer to eliminate them because, in practice, they are quite often a problem. Permitted foods include meat, fowl, fish, vegetables (including root vegetables), fruit, nuts, seeds, filtered or mineral water, herb teas and sea salt.

This diet is very limited, but usually reveals food sensitivities if they exist. It is normal for individuals to feel the benefit of this elimination diet after only five to ten days.

Overcoming food sensitivities

The first step in overcoming food sensitivities is to avoid the problem foodstuff(s). The question is, for how long? In normal circumstances, it is wise for problem foods to be excluded from the diet for a month. Two months is better, if you can manage it. There is no doubt that abstaining from a food for a period of time can make the body more tolerant to the food in the long term. Many individuals find that after about two months of wheat exclusion, they can go back to eating wheat without it having the adverse effects experienced before. However, with regard to food reintroduction, there are few things that need to be borne in mind:

1. For some time after a food is excluded from the diet, the body's reaction to it is often worse than it was before.

Even though exclusion of a food from the diet is ultimately likely to lead to greater tolerance of that food, it can take a month or two (or longer) for this to occur. In fact, for some time after the point of exclusion, it is common for an adverse reaction to a foodstuff to be worse than it was before. For example, while wheat may have caused problems with abdominal bloating and wind, reintroducing it again just a couple of weeks after it had been excluded may provoke bloating, wind, diarrhoea and abdominal discomfort. Experiencing a reaction of this nature might be quite alarming, but it can also help to reinforce the idea that the food is not the best thing for you to continue eating in the long term.

2. When a food is reintroduced, it is best not to eat too much of it, or too frequently.

It is usually possible to reintroduce a problem food back into the diet and not have any further problems with it. However, if that food is eaten in relatively large quantities and/or is eaten quite frequently, then this increases the risk of the original problems recurring. For instance, if you find that you have an intolerance of wheat, exclude it for a couple of months, and then go back to your regime of toast for breakfast, sandwich for lunch and pasta for the evening meal, you will almost certainly experience a recurrence of your original problems. However, if you confine yourself to the occasional sandwich or bowl of pasta, then your chances of further problems are much lower. In fact, when reintroducing problem foods it is a good idea to eat them in rotation. This means that you should only eat the food once every few days, often every three or four days. So, you can have toast for breakfast on Sunday, followed by a pasta supper on Wednesday, but, if you have no other wheat in between, it is unlikely to re-ignite the original weight or health problems that led you to exclude wheat in the first place.

As a general piece of advice about putting foods back into the diet, I say avoid it when you can and don't worry when you can't. In other words, avoid buying the foodstuffs that have been found to be a problem and opt for something else when choosing from a menu. However, if you're at a friend's house for dinner and pasta is being served, eat it, and for goodness sake don't let the fact that you're eating wheat ruin the meal for you.

3. In the long term, food sensitivities can be reduced by improving digestion and healing the lining of the gut.
Earlier in this chapter we discussed how poor digestion and leakiness in the intestinal wall could underlie a food sensitivity problem. Discerning whether or not these factors are, in fact, a problem, and combating them if they are, can really help to reduce the likelihood of old food sensitivities returning or new ones developing.

Improving digestion in the stomach

A healthy stomach contains acid for the digestion of protein-based foods such as meat, fish and eggs. One of the most common symptoms associated with some dysfunction in the stomach is indigestion. Traditionally, indigestion is often thought to be related to the over-production of acid in the stomach. This is why the conventional medical drugs prescribed for indigestion are essentially geared to reducing stomach acidity. However, for many, problems with indigestion stem from too *little* acid, not too much. A low level of acid in the stomach stalls the digestion of food, causing it to ferment. If you tend to suffer from bloating, belching or burning immediately after meals, feel that food tends to get stuck in the upper abdomen or that you only need to eat a small quantity to feel full, suspect low stomach acid.

Stomach acid isn't just important for the digestion of food, it also plays a critical role in the absorption of certain nutrients, including minerals such as iron and vitamins such as B12 and folic acid. All of these nutrients are essential for healthy red-blood-cell formation. As a result, long-standing low acid secretion can lead to a problem with anaemia. If you tend to be anaemic, and find that supplementation with iron or other nutrients is not really helping the condition, you need to consider the possibility of low stomach acid.

Apart from indigestion, other symptoms which suggest low acid secretion include weak nails and/or poor hair quality. Nails that are brittle or tend to flake and peel are quite common symptoms in women with low stomach acid. Men, even though their stomach acid secretion is low, tend not to suffer from weak nails. Another common symptom in women is hair that is thin, brittle and tends not to grow well. Interestingly, weak nails and poor hair quality tend not to coincide in an individual. It's usually one symptom or the other, but rarely both.

Low stomach acidity has also been associated with other illnesses, particularly those in which the body's immune system has turned against its own tissues (auto-immune diseases). Some of the conditions associated with low stomach acid, or that may point to this problem, include thyroid disease, eczema, gallbladder symptoms, osteoporosis, rheumatoid arthritis, chronic urticaria (hives), systemic lupus erythematosus (SLE, lupus), vitiligo (depigmentation of the skin) and rosacea (a facial skin disorder).

Medical tests for stomach acidity

Probably the most accurate medical test for stomach acidity is something called radiotelemetry. For this, the subject swallows a capsule on a thin piece of string. The capsule, known as a Heidelberg capsule, contains a pH-sensitive electrode. Once in the stomach, the capsule transmits a reading of the stomach acidity, which is detected by a sensing device held over the stomach on the skin's surface. This test is accurate and relatively inexpensive. However, it is not considered to be part of mainstream medicine, and your doctor may not have heard of it. For details on testing facilities, see the 'Useful Information' section at the back of the book under the name *Biolab*.

A home test for low stomach acid

While the radiotelemetry test described above can be a very good way to diagnose a low acid problem, a simple home test can help to identify this condition. Take a level teaspoon of bicarbonate of soda and dissolve it in some water. Drink this mixture on an empty stomach. If sufficient quantities of acid are present in the stomach, bicarbonate of soda is converted into gas, producing significant bloating and belching within five or ten minutes of drinking the mix. Little or no belching is suspicious for low stomach acid.

Problems with digestive enzymes

Another potential cause of poor digestion and food sensitivity is a lack of the digestive enzymes normally present in the small intestine. Some of these enzymes are naturally present in the lining of the digestive tract, but most are secreted by the pancreas and enter the small intestine via a small tube known as the pancreatic duct. Low levels of digestive enzymes can also provoke feelings of fullness after meals and symptoms such as indigestion, bloating, belching and wind. However, whereas individuals with low stomach acidity tend to experience their symptoms immediately after meals, those with an enzyme problem will usually start to get symptoms one to three hours after the meal.

Natural methods for improving digestion

Certain supplements can be used to improve digestion, and we will cover these at the end of the chapter. However, there's an enormous amount that can be done to improve the digestion before you reach for the supplement bottle.

1. Chew your food thoroughly

Proper chewing is essential for proper digestion. As mentioned earlier in this chapter, chewing stimulates the secretion of acid and digestive enzymes. Chewing also mixes food with saliva which contains an enzyme that starts the digestion of starchy foods such as bread, potatoes, rice and pasta. And, perhaps most importantly of all, chewing breaks food up, massively increasing the surface area available for contact with the digestive juices. This increases the efficiency of digestion by giving digestive enzymes the opportunity to penetrate the food and do the digestive work. Each mouthful should be chewed to a cream before swallowing.

2. Avoid big meals

The larger the meal is, the larger the load is on the digestive system. Small, frequent meals ease the burden on the digestive system and reduce the risk of indigestion.

3. Avoid drinking with meals

Some people tend to drink quite a lot of fluid with meals and it is widely believed that this helps to 'wash food down'. The reality is quite the reverse. Drinking with meals dilutes the acid and enzymes that do the digestive work, and so does nothing to help the process of digestion. For the main part, drinking should be done between meals, not at a mealtime.

4. Consider food combining

Foods are made up of several chemical constituents, including proteins, starches, fats, vitamins, minerals, fibre and water. The common proteins in the diet can be found in animal products such as meat, fish, dairy products and eggs. The common starches in the diet are bread, rice, pasta, cereals and potatoes. Proteins and starches are very different chemically and are digested by different enzymes in the gut. In addition, proteins are initially digested in acid, while starches are digested in alkali (quite the opposite). Some people find that their digestive systems are unable to cope with protein and starch at the same meal and this can lead to impaired digestion.

The principle of food-combining theory is to avoid mixing protein and starch at the same meal. This means eating either protein or starch, and combining it with a food which is classified as 'neutral' (neither protein nor starch). Eating to this pattern can bring tremendous relief to sufferers of indigestion and increase the chances of complete and rapid food breakdown.

The following list includes all the common protein, starch and neutral foods.

1. Protein

Meats:

bacon
beef
chicken
lamb
pork
turkey
veal
venison

Fish:
cod
herring
mackerel
plaice
salmon
skate
trout
tuna

Shellfish:
cockles
crab
lobster
mussels
oysters
prawns

Dairy products:
cheese
cream
eggs
milk
yoghurt

2. Neutral

All green and root vegetables apart from potatoes:
asparagus
aubergines
broccoli
Brussels sprouts
cabbage
carrots
cauliflower
celery
courgettes
green beans
leeks
mushrooms
onions
parsnips
peas
spinach
turnips

Salad vegetables:
avocado
cucumber
tomatoes
lettuce
spring onions
red and green peppers
radishes

Nuts and seeds
pumpkin
sunflower
sesame

3. Starch

bread
cereal
pasta
potato
rice

Foods made with flour:
biscuits
cakes
pastries & pies

Dried fruits:
currants
dates
figs
raisins
sultanas

Other fruit:
bananas
mangoes

Sweeteners:
honey
maple syrup
sugar

1. Protein	2. Neutral	3. Starch
Vegetable proteins:	**Nuts:**	
butter	almonds	
soya beans	cashews	
soya bean curd	peanuts	
(tofu)		
	Fats and oils:	
	butter	
	extra virgin olive oil	
	other vegetable oils	

So, according to the principles of food combining listed above, examples of healthy meals include:

> Meat or fish with salad, or vegetables other than potatoes
>
> Pasta with tomato-based sauce (no meat) and salad
>
> Vegetable curry and rice
>
> Baked potato, ratatouille and salad
>
> Meat stew with vegetables
>
> Avocado salad sandwich

Healing the gut lining

Leakiness in the gut wall (see page 91) may be an important factor in food sensitivity. It seems likely that problem foods may initiate immune reactions in the gut wall itself and that the inflammation caused by such reactions may lead to leakiness in the gut wall. This means that if gut leakiness is present, then excluding problem foods from the diet is very likely to help the gut lining to heal. If candida overgrowth is present (see chapter 7, *Break the Mould*), then clearing this is also very likely to help. However, it is also known that certain nutrients can contribute significantly to the health of the gut lining, so taking them in supplement form may help to heal the gut and prevent food sensitivities in the long term.

Supplements for overcoming food sensitivity

HCl and pepsin – supplements of HCl (hydrochloric acid) – taken in capsule form can certainly assist in the digestive process in individuals who have low or no stomach acid. Part of the action of hydrochloric acid is to convert an inactive substance called pepsinogen into an active enzyme called pepsin. The function of pepsin is to start the digestion of protein food molecules. Acid supplements are therefore best combined with pepsin for maximum potency. Acid supplements should be taken before meals.

Caution

Acid supplements should not be used if there is a present or past history or peptic ulcers (stomach and duodenum) or gastritis (inflammation of the stomach lining), unless under the instruction of a doctor with a bias towards nutrition.

Suggested supplement:

Acidol and pepsin – this combined supplement contains betaine hydrochloride (the type of acid most commonly used to acidify the stomach), along with pepsin. The normal recommended dose is one capsule, to be taken before each main meal. Acidol and Pepsin may be very effective in improving digestion and can often help to reduce the tendency to food sensitivity in time.

Availability

Details of how to obtain Acidol and Pepsin can be found in the section entitled 'Useful Information' section at the back of the book under the name *VitaTech*.

Digestive enzymes – digestive enzyme supplements may help to make up for inadequate or sub-optimal digestion in the small intestine. A good digestive enzyme supplement will normally contain a range of enzymes, each of which is responsible for digesting a certain food type. Examples of such enzymes include:

Protease – for the digestion of protein
Bromelain – for the digestion of protein
Amylase – for the digestion of starch
Sucrase – for the digestion of sugar (sucrose)
Cellulase – for the digestion of cellulose in plant matter
Lactase – for the digestion of lactose (milk sugar)

Lipase – for the digestion of fat

Maltase – for the digestion of maltose (a form of sugar found in some grains and made naturally in the gut)

Suggested Supplement:

Enzyme Forte – this is a combination supplement that contains the enzymes protease, bromelain, amylase, lipase, cellulase, lactase, sucrase and maltase. One capsule should be taken after each main meal. By helping to ensure the complete digestion of food, Enzyme Forte may help combat food sensitivities in the long term.

Contraindications

Enzyme Forte should not be used in individuals suffering from gastritis (inflammation of the stomach lining) or stomach/duodenal ulceration.

Availability

Details of how to obtain Enzyme Forte can be found in the section entitled 'Useful Information' section at the back of the book under the name *VitaTech*.

Gut healing nutrients – certain nutrients have an important role to play in healing the gut lining. Some of the important nutrients in this respect include:

Glutamine – an essential fuel for the cells which make up the lining of the small intestine, glutamine can help to promote healing in the gut.

N-acetyl glucosamine (NAG) – glucosamine is a nutrient known to help in the regeneration of body tissues. In its sulphate form it has been used traditionally to treat cartilage, ligament and tendon-related problems (e.g. osteoarthritis). However, in its N-acetyl form, it provides a sort of tissue cement to help bind gut cells together.

Gamma oryzanol – actually an extract of rice bran, gamma oryzanol has anti-inflammatory and healing properties within the gut.

Vitamin E and Vitamins A – both of these nutrients play an important role in gut lining healing.

Suggested Supplement:

Permaguard – a combination supplement which contains L-glutamine, N-acetyl glucosamine, gamma oryzanol, vitamin E, vitamin A and the healthy gut organism L. acidophilus. Long-term supplementation with Permaguard may promote healing in the lining of the digestive tract, reducing the risk of food sensitivity. The recommended dose is one capsule, three times a day.

Availability

Details of how to obtain Permaguard can be found in the 'Useful Information' section at the back of the book under the name *VitaTech*.

Case Study

Joanne B is a 27-year-old housewife and mother of three

> *I have had a variety of health problems since my late teens. While I was still at school I developed all sorts of digestive problems including bloating, wind and constipation. Over the years I had noticed that I would get tired for no obvious reason, especially after meals. Sometimes I would just feel completely drained. I used to exercise a lot, but since having the kids I just haven't had the time. I've always been a little on the large size, but in recent years I've really begun to pile of the pounds. Just over a year ago I weighed 11 stones 10 pounds. I really wanted to be 9½ stones, but eating sensibly would only take off a few pounds which I'd put back on anyway.*
>
> *For some time, I had suspected I might have a problem with certain foods, so I booked an appointment with a natural practitioner. The test (electro-dermal testing) revealed that I had a problem with wheat, milk, coffee and wine. I remember walking out from my appointment thinking how much sense this all made. I had always eaten a high wheat bran breakfast cereal (my doctor told me this would help my irritable bowel syndrome) with milk for breakfast, would invariably eat a sandwich for*

lunch, and had several cups of coffee with milk each day. Maybe twice a week I would eat pasta for my evening meal, and I would have a glass or two of wine most evenings. No wonder I was having problems!

A couple of days later I started the elimination diet. I had rye toast and egg, or corn- or rice-based cereal with rice milk for breakfast. I had a salad for lunch, maybe with some rye crackers. Supper was meat or fish with vegetables. I didn't feel the effects for a few days. However, I remember distinctly on the fourth day of the diet feeling so much more alive. My fatigue after meals had gone and I just felt lighter. The weight started to shift almost right away. In the first two weeks I lost 8 pounds. I continued losing weight and eventually got down to 10 stones in about five or six months. Another fantastic benefit from all of this was that my irritable bowel syndrome all but disappeared.

From time to time I will eat wheat and drink wine, usually if I'm out at a dinner party or something. As long as I don't push it, I'm fine. I no longer drink coffee or milk and am into peppermint tea now. Sometimes people ask me if I miss eating bread and pasta. If they knew just how much better I feel not having it, I don't think they'd ever bother asking.

Summary

- Food sensitivity is an important, and often undiagnosed, cause of weight gain and ill-health.

- Food sensitivity is often related to problems with poor digestion or leakiness in the digestive tract.

- Traditional methods of food testing (IgE blood tests and scratch tests) are not appropriate for diagnosing the types of food reactions that lead to weight gain and long-term illness.

- Methods which can be used to diagnose food sensitivities include elimination dieting, blood tests (cytotoxic, ALCAT, IgG), electro-dermal testing and applied kinesiology.

- Foodstuffs which have been identified as a problem should be eliminated from the diet for one to two months, after which time they can often be reintroduced in small amounts without causing a recurrence of the original symptoms.

- Taking measures to improve digestion and reduce leakiness in the gut wall is likely to reduce the risk of food sensitivity in the long term.

- Successfully dealing with a food sensitivity problem can lead to significant weight loss and improved well-being.

CHAPTER 7

Break the Mould

D o you suffer from irritable bowel syndrome? Is abdominal bloating and/or wind a problem for you? Do you tend to get thrush (vaginal yeast infection) from time to time? Does your energy level tend to fluctuate during the day? Do you often crave sweet or starchy foods? Do you suffer from recurrent cystitis (urinary tract infection)? Do you tend to suffer from episodes of fuzzy headedness, poor memory and lapses in concentration? Do you find it almost impossible to lose weight, even when you cut back on food? Do you have a lot of mystery symptoms that you're finding it difficult to get to the bottom of?

If you identify with some, or all, of the above symptoms and scenarios, then it is quite likely that there is an overgrowth of yeast in your body. This chapter concerns itself with the yeast organism, *Candida albicans*, and the role it can play in problems related to weight and health. Candida albicans, which we'll refer to as candida from here on in, lives in pretty much everyone's intestinal tract and, for the most part, doesn't create any problems. However, under certain circumstances candida has the capacity to overgrow in the gut, which may in turn lead to a vast array of potential symptoms. What is more, any practitioner who has treated this condition will tell you that some of the most profound changes in health happen in individuals who successfully tackle their yeast problem.

Yeast overgrowth is a contentious issue. While it is well-accepted as a very real problem by many natural health practitioners, conventional doctors are usually more sceptical. I remember learning about candida at medical school. The sorts of problems attributed to this organism were essentially confined to relatively minor manifestations such as candida in the mouth and vaginal yeast infections, or terrible overwhelming infections most commonly seen in those with terminal cancer or advanced HIV infection. Curiously, though, there did not seem to be any mention of candida between these two extremes. More naturally-oriented practitioners have come to recognize that candida in the body can give rise to a whole spectrum of health problems, which extend far beyond those recognized by most doctors.

The internal ecosystem

The main components of the gut are the mouth (where the digestion of starches starts), stomach (where the digestion of protein starts), small intestine (where fats, proteins and starches are digested and absorbed) and large intestine (where water is absorbed and from which waste matter is eliminated). The gut is by no means a sterile environment. Actually, it's packed with bacteria. The word bacteria generally conjures up negative images. We all know that bacteria are responsible for infections. They are often at the root of problems such as cystitis, chest infections and meningitis. However, for the main part, the bacteria in the gut are actually healthy, and they participate in a number of beneficial body processes. Each of us holds about one and a half kilograms (three or four pounds) of bacteria in our intestinal tracts, and several important roles have been identified for them.

1. Enhanced food digestion and absorption

Milk contains a sugar called lactose, which is digested by an enzyme called lactase in the small intestine. Some individuals, especially those of black, Asian and southern European heritage, lack the ability to digest lactose efficiently. This problem, which is referred to as lactose intolerance, can lead to problems which include abdominal bloating and discomfort, excessive flatulence and loose stools.

Lactobacillus acidophilus (one of the principle organisms in the small intestine) has the ability to enhance lactose digestion, and may therefore improve symptoms in individuals who are prone to lactose intolerance.

2. Protecting the gut from unhealthy organisms

The healthy gut bacteria also protect the gut from infection or overgrowth of unhealthy organisms such as yeast, parasites and unwanted bacteria. The healthy bacteria do this in a number of ways, which include crowding out unwanted organisms (1), making the gut more acidic and therefore more hostile to unwanted organisms (2) and by producing antibiotic-like substances (3).

3. Reducing the amount of cholesterol in the body

Supplementation with Lactobacillus acidophilus or Lactobacillus acidophilus-containing food products (e.g. live yoghurt) appears to have the ability to reduce the level of cholesterol in the bloodstream (4).

4. Immune system activation

There is some evidence that certain species of healthy bacteria have been found to stimulate the immune system directly, enhancing the production of an important immune chemical, beta-interferon (5).

So, we can see that the healthy gut bacteria have an important part to play in maintaining health, both inside and outside the gut. Later on, we'll be discussing how the loss of healthy gut bacteria may contribute to the overgrowth of candida, and how to restore healthy bacterial balance through dietary change and the use of nutritional supplements.

The healthy gut and what can go wrong

A healthy gut tends to contain relatively large amounts of healthy bacterial species and little in the way of yeast. As long as the balance of gut organisms is towards the beneficial bacteria, then that's O.K. It's only when yeast overgrows and/or healthy bacterial species are lost in significant numbers that problems can perhaps arise, (see diagram overleaf). The factors which may encourage an imbalance in the intestinal ecosystem include:

1. Antibiotics

Antibiotics are a major, perhaps *the* most important, factor in candida overgrowth. Designed to kill harmful bacteria in the body, most antibiotics are taken by mouth. Down in the gut, antibiotics have the capacity to cut a swathe through the healthy gut bacteria, but do not touch yeast. As a result, antibiotics can lead to a predominance of yeast in the gut. Some women find that they can be prone to a vaginal yeast infection (thrush) if they take antibiotics. The killing of healthy gut bacteria by antibiotics, and subsequent yeast overgrowth explains this phenomenon.

In practice, antibiotics are very often at the root of an individual's candida problem. Quite commonly the imbalance is created way back in childhood or adolescence. What seems to happen frequently is that the individual starts with some form of food sensitivity, often milk, at a young age. Milk sensitivity will quite often give rise to problems with ear infections, tonsillitis, sinusitis and the like. Multiple courses of antibiotics will usually be prescribed for these problems, which in turn sows the seeds for a candida problem later in life. Medium- and long-term antibiotics prescribed to cure acne can also set up a significant imbalance and this is another common scenario for candida sufferers.

The intestinal ecosystem

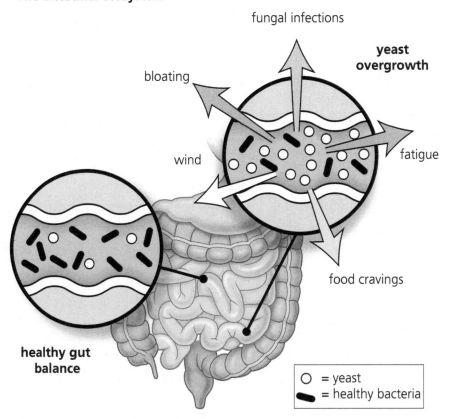

2. Stress

Stress is a common and important feature in so many people's lives. It has been shown to reduce immune activity, with the potential result that organisms such as candida can escape the body's normal control mechanisms and grow out of control in the gut and elsewhere in the body.

Stress is also known to have a number of direct effects on the gut itself, including a reduction in certain secretions that are normally present and changes in the time it takes for food to pass along the gut. It is possible that these factors may also precipitate the growth of yeast in the gut.

3. Diet

Yeast is a living organism and it thrives on certain foods that provide ready fuel for the yeast cells. Foods which encourage yeast growth in this way include sugar and refined carbohydrates such as white-flour products, pasta and white rice. Other foods that encourage yeast growth include those that are yeasty, mouldy or fermented in their own right such as bread, alcohol, mushrooms, yeast-extract spread, peanuts, pistachios, dried fruit, vinegar and soy sauce (see pages 122–130). The preponderance of yeast-encouraging foods in the average modern Western diet may help to explain the apparent prevalence of candida and the problems which are associated with it.

4. The Pill and HRT

It is generally noted that candida overgrowth is a more common problem in women than in men. This is thought to be due, at least in part, to the presence of female hormones such as oestrogen and progesterone and their effect on yeast production. The presence of these hormones in significant quantities appears to encourage yeast growth in the body. The oral contraceptive pill and hormone replacement therapy (HRT) are both based on female hormones. Taking them is therefore thought to encourage candida proliferation in the body.

Is candida your problem?

The following questionnaire is designed to help you ascertain whether there is an overgrowth of yeast in your body. Score each question as indicated and then add up your total score.

1. Do you suffer from significant abdominal bloating?

No –   0 points
Occasional or mild problems – 2 points
Frequent or severe problems – 4 points

2. Do you suffer from anal itching?

No –   0 points
Occasional or mild problems – 2 points
Frequent or severe problems – 4 points

3. Do you find that your bowel habit can be somewhat erratic, perhaps constipated some of the time and loose at others?

No –   0 points
Occasional or mild problems – 2 points
Frequent or severe problems – 4 points

4. Do you tend to suffer from excessive wind and flatulence?

No –   0 points
Occasional or mild problems – 2 points
Frequent or severe problems – 4 points

5. Do you suffer from thrush (vaginal yeast infection) from time to time?

No –   0 points
Occasional or mild problems – 3 points
Frequent or severe problems – 6 points

6. Do you suffer from pre-menstrual syndrome or painful or irregular periods?

No –   0 points
Occasional or mild problems – 1 points
Frequent or severe problems – 2 points

7. Do you suffer from episodes of mental confusion, mental fatigue, loss of concentration, low mood or irritability?

No –   0 points
Occasional or mild problems – 2 points
Frequent or severe problems – 4 points

8. Do you suffer from periodic skin problems such as urticaria (hives), athlete's foot, generalized itching or a rash between your buttocks or in your groin?

No –   0 points
Occasional or mild problems – 3 points
Frequent or severe problems – 6 points

9. Do you suffer from recurrent bouts of cystitis and/or problems with vaginal irritation?

No –   0 points
Occasional or mild problems – 3 points
Frequent or severe problems – 5 points

10. Do you crave sugar, sugary foods such as chocolate, biscuits or cakes, or yeasty foods such as cheese, bread, alcohol or vinegar?

No –   0 points
Occasional or mild problems – 2 points
Frequent or severe problems – 4 points

11. Do you suffer from multiple allergies and react to chemicals in the environment such as petrol and diesel fumes, cleaning fluids and perfumes?

No –   0 points
Occasional or mild problems – 2 points
Frequent or severe problems – 4 points

12. How would you describe your antibiotic consumption in the past, including childhood?

Very few antibiotics generally –   0 points
Moderate use for occasional infections such
as winter infections, chest infections etc –   5 points
Frequent and/or extended use for problems
such as acne, recurrent urinary tract infections,
chronic sinusitis, tonsillitis, etc –   10 points

13. Have you currently been taking the oral contraceptive pill for more than six months or did you take it in the past for more than a year?

Yes –   3 points
No –   0 points

14. Have you had steroid drugs such as prednisolone, dexamethasone or betamethasone by mouth or cortisone injections?

Yes –   4 points
No –   0 points

15. Have you ever had inhaled steroids (usually for asthma) such as Becotide for three months or more?

Yes –   4 points
No –   0 points

16. Do you have a number of vague health problems no one has been able to explain?

Yes –   4 points
No –   0 points

Interpreting your score

0 – 9:   yeast overgrowth is unlikely
10 – 24:   yeast overgrowth should be considered as a possibility and further testing or a trial of the anti-candida regime is likely to be worthwhile
25 – 39:   yeast overgrowth is likely, and steps taken to combat yeast are very likely to help improve weight loss and general health
40 and above: yeast overgrowth is very likely, and steps taken to combat this are almost certainly going to improve weight loss and general health

If you have scored highly or moderately on the questionnaire, you may wish to confirm whether or not you have a yeast problem with some form of testing. Several types of tests are available, and the most commonly available are listed here:

Tests for candida

1. Yeast cultures

Stool samples and swabs taken from the vagina, mouth, throat or skin can be sent to a microbiological laboratory for yeast analysis. These tests generally need to be administrated by a doctor – and they are by no means foolproof. I don't think it's uncommon for someone with a genuine yeast problem (as indicated by their symptoms and response to treatment) to have his or her culture tests come up as clear. My tendency is to treat candida if the culture shows candida, but not necessarily discount candida if the test is normal.

2. Candida antigen in the blood

An antigen is a particle that stimulates the immune system. There is a specific blood test for candida antigen and, if this is positive, it probably indicates an ongoing yeast infection. Not only that, it also suggests that the yeast has escaped from the gut itself and has made its way into the bloodstream. Antigen tests are thought to provide pretty hard evidence of a candida infection, but there is always the possibility that if candida is confined to the gut, the blood test will be negative.

3. Candida antibodies in the blood

Antibodies are what the immune system produces in response to antigens. Two types of antibody, IgG and IgM, are usually measured. If the level of antibodies specific for candida is raised, this may indicate infection.

4. Candida antibodies in the gut

A type of antibody known as secretory IgA is produced within the gut. Measuring the amount of secretory IgA made specifically against candida can be a good guide to the presence of yeast in the gut. The higher the value, the more likely there is to be a yeast overgrowth in the intestine.

5. The gut fermentation test

Yeast tends to metabolize sugar into alcohol. The gut fermentation test is based on this principle. A blood sample is taken and the subject is then given a measured dose of sugar. An hour later, another sample of blood is taken. Both blood samples are analysed for various fermentation products. The presence of these substances in significant quantities can point to the presence of excess yeast in the gut.

6. Other tests

It is possible to diagnose yeast overgrowth through a number of non-laboratory tests, including iridology, electro-dermal testing (e.g. Vega, BEST system, Eclosion), dowsing and applied kinesiology. All of these forms of testing have their own merits, especially if the assessment is carried out by an experienced and skilled practitioner. Assessment is usually relatively cheap and the results are immediate. Another advantage with these forms of testing is that they invariably allow contact with a practitioner, who is likely to be able to guide you through the intricacies of an anti-candida programme if testing shows this to be a problem.

How important is testing for candida?

The short answer to this is, in my opinion, not much. I do think it is usually possible to diagnose candida by looking carefully for the symptoms and underlying factors that are typical in the condition. Occasionally, I may perform a test where the diagnosis really is questionable, but usually the patient's story gives it away.

Candida and food sensitivity

Anyone who has a significant yeast overgrowth in the gut will be prone to food sensitivity. It does appear that once yeast gets to a certain level, it has the ability to make the gut 'leaky'. The lining of the gut is really designed to allow the transit of very small food particles, which are then burnt for fuel, stored for later use or converted into some other body component such as muscle or a hormone. When the gut becomes leaky, it is possible that larger than desirable food particles can escape through the gut wall into the bloodstream, where they may provoke adverse reactions (see diagram opposite). These in turn may give rise to all sorts of symptoms, including weight gain, fatigue, fluid retention, eczema, migraine and inflammatory arthritis. (See chapter 6, *Eliminate your Allergies*).

So, by making the gut leakier than it should be, candida can contribute directly to problems with food sensitivity. Candida is also thought to impair digestion. So now we have a real double-whammy: inadequate digestion of food (meaning large food

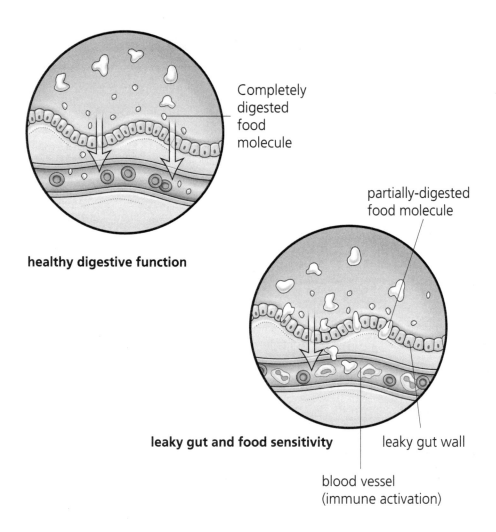

Completely digested food molecule

healthy digestive function

partially-digested food molecule

leaky gut and food sensitivity

leaky gut wall

blood vessel (immune activation)

particles in the gut) coupled with a greater risk of these food particles getting into the system. Experience shows that candida sufferers usually have some food sensitivities, and it appears that continuing to eat these foods tends to delay recovery from candida, even though the basic anti-candida diet is adhered to. For some, it may be appropriate to identify their food sensitivities using one or more of the techniques outlined in chapter 6. However, there is an easier way. Because sensitivities to dairy products and wheat are so common, it is wise to start by taking these two food types out of the diet. My feeling is that for the vast majority of people, a dairy and wheat-free, anti-candida diet is usually very effective in restoring health to the gut, even if there are one or more additional food sensitivities lurking that have not been identified or countered. The main wheat-containing and dairy foods that you should be aware of are covered later on in this chapter, along with some suggestions for viable alternatives.

The anti-candida diet

The cornerstone of the anti-candida approach is a diet that helps to starve yeast out of the system. This means eating no foods which feed yeast directly, or encourage yeast by being yeasty, mouldy or fermented in their own right.

Yeast-feeding foods to avoid

Sugar

Sweetening agents, such as maple syrup, molasses, honey and malt syrup

Sugar containing foods such as biscuits, cakes, confectionery, ice cream, pastries, sugared breakfast cereals, soft drinks and fruit juice

White flour products, including white bread, crackers, pizza and pasta

Yeasty, mouldy or fermented foods to avoid

Bread and other yeast-raised items

Alcoholic drinks, particularly beer and wine which are very yeasty

Gravy mixes (most contain brewer's yeast)

Vinegar and vinegar-containing foods, such as tomato ketchup (which also contains sugar), mustard, mayonnaise and many prepared salad dressings

Pickles, miso, tempeh and soy sauce (all fermented)

Aged cheeses including cheddar, stilton, Swiss, brie and camembert (cheese is inherently mouldy)

Peanuts (and peanut butter) and pistachios (which tend to harbour yeast)

Mushrooms (mushrooms are mould!)

Dried fruit (these are intensely sugary and tend to harbour mould)

Yeast-containing foods such as soups and pre-packaged foods

As we mentioned earlier, individuals who have a candida problem are likely to be sensitive to wheat and/or dairy products. The safest bet is also to avoid these foods, at least for a month or two.

Wheat-containing foods to avoid

- Wheat bread (beware also of breads labelled as 'rye bread' which may also contain wheat flour – always check the labels)
- Wheat-based crackers
- Biscuits
- Pizza
- Cake
- Wheat-based breakfast cereals
- Pastry
- Anything containing wheat flour, including sauces and soups
- Breaded food
- Battered food

Dairy foods to avoid

Within the dairy food group it is really milk and cheese that tend to create the problems for sufferers of yeast overgrowth. Butter is usually very well tolerated, and natural, live, unsweetened yoghurt is usually O.K, too. Yoghurt also has the advantage of containing bacterial species (this is what the word 'live' refers to) that may contribute to the health of the gut. Soya milk and rice milk make good alternatives to cow's milk and can be drunk freely.

As you can see, there's a lot of foods that may need to be avoided on an anti-candida diet, the question is, what can you eat?

Foods to eat freely

The foods that are generally suitable to eat freely on an anti-candida regime are listed below:

Protein foods

Beef	Broccoli
Chicken	Brussels sprouts
Eggs	Cabbage
Duck	Cauliflower
Fish including naturally	Celery
smoked fish	Chard
Lamb	Cucumber
Pork	Green beans
Shellfish	Kale
Tofu (soya bean curd)	Leek
Turkey	Lettuce
Vegetables	Onion
Artichoke	Parsnips
Asparagus	Spinach
Aubergine	Tomato
Avocado	Watercress

Foods to be eaten in moderation

Certain foods, such as grains, high-starch vegetables, legumes or pulses, can be eaten on an anti-candida regime, but it's best not to eat masses of them as they do tend to have some fermentation potential. The bulk of the diet should be based around the foods which can be eaten freely, supplemented with more limited amounts of the foods that follow in this list:

High-starch vegetables

Potatoes

Squash (e.g. butternut)

Sweet potatoes

Legumes

Adzuki beans	Corn
Black beans	Millet
Kidney beans	Oats, oat cakes and
Lentils	oat-based breakfast
Lima beans	cereals
Navy beans	Quinoa
Split peas	Rice cakes
	Rye
Grains	Rye crackers
Barley	Wild rice
Brown rice	Spelt
Brown rice cakes	Yeast-free rye bread
Buckwheat	

What about fruit?

And finally, a word about fruit. Whether or not fruit is advisable on an anti-candida regime is a real moot point. Some practitioners say it can be eaten freely; others say it should be completely excluded, at least to begin with. I have to say, I take the middle ground. My experience is that one or two pieces of fruit a day is generally very well tolerated, though I'm no fan of grapes as they are usually intensely sugary and covered in a mouldy bloom. All fruit that you're not going to peel prior to eating should be washed thoroughly. The best fruits are those that contain the least sugar (raspberries, blueberries, grapefruit and fresh figs). Dried fruits, as mentioned before, are definitely off the menu for a while.

Candida and blood-sugar balance

The body likes to keep the level of sugar in the bloodstream between relatively narrow parameters, not too high, not too low. However, in certain individuals, the blood-sugar level can tend to fluctuate, and this can lead to symptoms such as fluctuating energy, cravings for sweet or starchy foods and problems with low mood, irritability or mood swings.

The food craving problem often experienced by candida sufferers can really scupper them. The cravings most individuals get on an anti-candida regime are usually for the foods that are worst for them. So, getting on top of a blood-sugar problem is of prime importance if the anti-candida diet is to be adhered to without too much angst. So, if you suffer from one or more of these symptoms, it will almost certainly help you to refer to chapter 3, *Balance your Blood Sugar*, which explains the principles of the blood-sugar stabilizing diet. In particular, the chapter also includes details of nutrients and supplements which may really help to counter this problem.

The anti-candida diet – quite a lot to think about

It is clear that in constructing an anti-candida diet, we often have to combine several approaches. Just to recap, the main principles are these:

1. Avoid foods and drinks which feed yeast (sugar and refined carbohydrates)

2. Avoid food and drinks which encourage yeast (yeasty, mouldy or fermented foods).

3. Avoid wheat, milk and cheese as these foods are common sensitivities in candida sufferers (cheese also tends to encourage yeast overgrowth).

4. Eat a diet based on foods which release sugar slowly into the bloodstream.

Now, if you add to these principles the fact that the diet should be essentially healthy and acceptable to you, what does this leave? What I've outlined below is a few menu suggestions to help you get on your way. I'm well aware that I do not know your dietary preferences but, in my experience, just about everyone will find foods within these suggestions that are practical and palatable. Here goes:

Breakfast

Oats (soaked overnight in water or milk substitute) with chopped almonds and hazelnuts, pumpkin and sunflower seeds, rice or soya milk, natural, live unsweetened yoghurt and some chopped fresh fruit

Oat porridge made with water, soya or rice milk, sweetened with banana

Puffed brown rice cereal, or non-wheat multi-grain cereal (HFS) with rice or soya milk, natural yoghurt, nuts, seeds and some fruit.

Poached egg on yeast-free rye-bread toast

Kipper or haddock with poached egg, grilled tomatoes and yeast-free rye-bread toast

Lunch and supper

Brown-rice salad (brown rice with a variety of added ingredients such as tuna, chicken, chick peas, tomato, bell peppers, cucumber, spring onion, garlic and herbs, with a dressing made from extra virgin olive oil and lemon juice)

Chicken or tuna salad sandwich made with yeast-free rye bread

Chicken, tuna or prawn salad (with an extra virgin olive oil and lemon juice dressing) with rye crackers or brown-rice cakes

Spanish omelette (without cheese) and salad

Poached salmon with steamed vegetables and a few boiled new potatoes

Grilled chicken and roast vegetables, including some potato

Chicken, turkey or fish with brown rice and salad

Stir-fried tofu and vegetables with brown rice or rice noodles

The supplements

I can't stress strongly enough how important the anti-candida diet is to overcoming a candida problem. There really is no point in swallowing handfuls of supplements if your diet is full of bread, cheese and wine. However, in conjunction with a good diet, certain supplements really do seem to be able to speed recovery and restore health to the gut and the body. The basic nutritional supplements often used to accompany an anti-candida programme include the following:

1. Healthy gut bacteria supplements to restore the intestinal ecosystem

2. Liver-supporting agents to protect the liver and the rest of the body from the toxins that can be released during the initial phase of an anti-candida regime

3. Nutrients to support blood-sugar stability

4. Supplements to kill yeast

5. Supplements to help heal the gut lining

Not all of these need be used in every individual. In my experience, the first three play a big role in the management of the vast majority of sufferers, while the last two types of supplements seem to be required less.

1. Healthy gut bacteria supplements

Healthy gut bacteria supplements are also known as 'probiotics' because they put bacteria back into the body; the opposite of antibiotics, which take them away. It has been claimed that often the supplements that are bought in health food stores do not contain what they say they contain. There is some evidence to show that some supplements do not contain the quantities of living organisms declared on the label, and some claim to contain organisms which shouldn't be there. If you know of a reputable brand of probiotics, that's fine. If you don't, I've listed a couple of suitable probiotics here.

Replant – a probiotic supplement that adds massive numbers of healthy bacteria into the gut. It is particularly useful in the initial stages of an anti-candida regime. Taken at this time, I have noticed that it can significantly speed recovery from yeast and the re-establishment of healthy gut organisms. Replant contains three organisms:

Lactobacillus acidophilus – the predominant organism in the small intestine

Bifidobacterium bifidus – the predominant organism in the large intestine

Lactobacillus bulgaricus – an organism which has been linked with health and well-being in individuals who consume yoghurt rich in this organism

Replant comes in sachets, each of which provides thirty million organisms (ten million of each organism). The supplement should be taken for a week, and I generally recommend that half a sachet is taken twice a day.

Replant very often causes increased bloating and wind, and very occasionally discomfort. These symptoms may be caused by a war going on between the healthy gut bacteria and the less healthy organisms, including yeast. The symptoms normally only last for three or four days and are usually very manageable.

Acidophilus forte – is a probiotic supplement suitable for continued use. It contains a combination of lactobacillus acidophilus and bifidobacterium bifidus.The total dose of organisms per capsule is six billion – a good dose of healthy gut bacteria in the initial stages of an anti-candida regime if taken twice a day.

Availability
Details of how to obtain Replant and Acidophilus Forte can be found in the 'Useful Information' section at the back of the book under the name *VitaTech*.

2. Liver support
During the initial phases of an anti-candida regime, it is quite common for individuals to experience a worsening in their condition. Symptoms such as lethargy, fuzzy-headedness and flu-like symptoms can start a day or so after the regime starts. The symptoms generally last from between a few days to a couple of weeks. This reaction is sometimes referred to a 'die-off', and is thought to be due to an increase in

candida-derived toxins in the system. If yeast cells die, they will tend to liberate toxic substances that pass from the gut to the liver. Often, the liver does not cope adequately with them, which can allow the toxins to escape into the circulation, where they may give rise to the sort of symptoms listed above.

One way to help reduce the effects of die-off is to use liver-supporting agents. Certain herbs and nutrients have the ability to strengthen the detoxifying action of the liver, which in turn can increase the likelihood of toxins being neutralized effectively in the liver before they get the chance to get into the bloodstream. (For a list of some of the main liver-supporting agents and a combination supplement which may help protect the liver during the initial phases of an anti-candida regime are covered see chapter 8, *Keep it Clean*.)

3. Blood sugar control

If you exhibit symptoms of blood-sugar imbalance, and particularly if food cravings are a problem, you may well benefit from taking nutrients that play a role in maintaining blood-sugar levels. (For a list of these nutrients and a suitable combination supplement see chapter 3, *Balance Your Blood Sugar*).

4. Anti-fungal supplements

Some of the natural agents which may be useful in combating yeast in the body include:

Oregano – this has been employed as an antiseptic in herbal and folk medicine for thousands of years. Oregano contains a number of active ingredients, probably the two most important of which are carvacrol and thymol. Studies have shown that oregano has anti-fungal properties and can inhibit the growth of candida.

Garlic – like oregano, garlic has a tradition of use in herbal medicine that goes back thousands of years. Garlic has the ability to kill a range of organisms, including bacteria, viruses, parasites and fungi. In natural medicine, garlic is a widely used substance in the control and eradication of candida.

Grapefruit seed extract – this is thought to have the ability to kill candida in the body. Many sufferers report that taking grapefruit-seed extract has helped them to control their symptoms and conquer their yeast-related problems.

Suggested Supplement:
Canditrol – this combination supplement has been specifically formulated to combat yeast in the body. It contains garlic, oregano oil and grapefruit-seed extract. If I do recommend an anti-fungal supplement, I normally advise that it is taken for three or four months, starting a month after the anti-candida diet is commenced. The normal recommended dose for Canditrol is one capsule with food, twice a day.

NOTE: Canditrol capsules should not be chewed or opened.

Contraindications
Canditrol should not be used during pregnancy or if pregnancy is planned. The use of Canditrol should also be avoided in cases of gastritis (inflammation of the stomach lining) and stomach/duodenal ulceration.

Availability
Details of how to obtain Canditrol can be found in the 'Useful Information' section at the back of the book under the name *VitaTech*.

5. Gut healing nutrients
For a list of the nutrients thought to play an important part in healing and soothing the lining of the gut, and the recommendation of a specific supplement, see chapter 6, *Eliminate Your Allergies*.

A suggested protocol for anti-candida supplements – while each individual with a candida problem may have their own requirements, in my experience, the vast majority do well by starting their supplement regime using probiotics, along with supplements to support liver function and blood-sugar levels. If an anti-fungal supplement is to be used, then this is usually best added after a month of treatment. Adding it earlier may lead to large numbers of yeast cells dying at once, increasing the risk of 'die-off'. If it seems appropriate to use a gut healing agent, then this might be added a month after the anti-fungal supplement is started.

In mild cases of candida, there is usually no need to progress to anti-fungal and gut healing supplemnts, and a good diet supported by the basic supplements for three or four months is likely to be enough. In more severe cases, anti-fungal and gut healing supplements have more of a role to play, and treatment tends to be longer – often six to twelve months. It may help you, particularly if your problem is severe, to work with a practitioner experienced in candida related problems.

Case Study

Katherine P is a 35-year-old shoe designer

> *For years I had been suffering with more health problems than I care to mention. I suppose my main problem was irritable bowel syndrome. I first started noticing problems with bloating and discomfort when I was about 14 years old. I lost count of the number of tests I'd had for this. After five years of investigations, I was prescribed tablets, which didn't work, and told to eat plenty of bran, which made things worse.*
>
> *My skin had also been a problem since my late teens. I'd tried the usual stuff, lotions and potions and what have you, but eventually I took a course of antibiotics. These controlled my skin problem, but the problem just came back after I stopped them. I ended up taking some dreadful drug, but had to stop due to side-effects.*
>
> *Going back, I remember not being well as a child. I had tonsillitis from about the age of five to when I was seven. My mother told me that one time I was given four lots of antibiotics in as many months. Eventually they took my tonsils out when I was seven, but I never really felt well after this.*
>
> *Another main issue that I had was my weight. I think the weight had been steadily going on since I was a girl. I was a bit on the chubby side, but had grown into a fully-fledged size 16 as the years went by. No amount of dieting really seemed to touch this problem. I found it difficult to control my diet. Quite often, I would get these powerful, uncontrollable urges to eat chocolate or biscuits. I felt very guilty about these binges, and*

guilty about not taking any exercise, too. I was in a right mess.

Two years ago, I decided to do something about my spiralling health problems and booked an appointment to see a nutritionist. I really wanted help to lose weight. I just didn't know what to eat. My practitioner seemed to know straight away what my problem was. She explained to me about candida and the problems it can produce. She also talked to me about my blood sugar. I was gripped. Suddenly, it all started to become clear why I'd been suffering all these years. I went on an anti-candida diet and eliminated wheat from my diet, too. I started on a bunch of supplements as well: healthy bacteria for my gut, something for my liver and something to help balance my blood sugar.

Even within a month, I was beginning to feel better. I had more energy and my irritable bowel was so much better. I hardly had any bloating, and my bowel habit started to regularize. I had more energy and my food cravings had just vanished. My skin was much clearer, too and, best of all, I'd lost weight. In just over a month I had lost ten pounds. Suddenly, I was able to get into clothes I hadn't worn for two years and I was thrilled.

After a couple of months on the diet my practitioner advised me to start relaxing things a bit. I also started to tail off the supplements. The whole thing took about five months. I've had a few problems from time to time, usually if I eat something like bread or pasta. Otherwise, I tend to be OK. I lost almost two stones in all, and my weight has stayed down. Physically and emotionally, I'm a different person to how I was a couple of years ago.

Summary

● Candida albicans is a yeast organism that inhabits the human gut.

● If candida overgrows in the gut it can lead to a wide range of health problems, including weight gain, irritable bowel syndrome, mood disturbance, fatigue and food cravings.

● Factors which encourage candida overgrowth include antibiotic use, stress, hormonal treatments and a diet containing foodstuffs that encourage yeast growth, including sugar, refined carbohydrates, bread and alcohol.

● Food sensitivity, particularly to wheat, milk and cheese, is often a feature in candida.

● Blood-sugar fluctuation is often a feature in candida, too.

● The cornerstone of the anti-candida regime is a diet which is based on foods that do not encourage candida growth.

● Supplements which help restore healthy gut bacteria can be very useful in the management of candida.

● Other supplements which are very often of use in managing candida are those that support the liver and help to stabilize the blood-sugar level.

● Natural anti-fungal supplements, and those that help heal the lining of the gut, may also be of benefit.

● Overcoming a yeast overgrowth problem and restoring health to the gut can be a very effective way of losing weight and combating a wide range of symptoms and conditions.

CHAPTER 8

Keep it Clean

'Toxin' is one of the buzzwords of natural health, and 'detox' diets seem to be everywhere. Speak to just about any practitioner of complementary medicine about health, and the subject of toxicity is almost sure to crop up somewhere. Toxins in the body are believed to be responsible for a whole host of symptoms and conditions, including weight gain, fatigue, bad breath and cellulite. The fact is, reducing the toxic load on the body, or getting the body to deal with toxins more effectively, can be a critical step towards losing weight and enhancing well-being.

Our toxic environment

Our body is constantly exposed to a stream of substances that can lead to toxicity within it. Some of these, such as the pollutants we breathe and the herbicides and pesticides that lace many of the foods we eat, come from the outside. Others are the result of the metabolic and physiological processes that go on in our bodies every day. The body has evolved ways to process and eliminate unwanted substances from the body. Unfortunately, partly due to the fact that we are now exposed to thousands of toxic substances from our environment, including those in our food supply, our body-cleansing processes can't always keep up. If the toxic load in the system is large, and/or if there is some problem with the body's detoxification processes, then toxins may build up. This toxic accumulation effectively poisons the body, and may manifest itself in a number of ways. As we have already mentioned, weight gain is one potential consequence of toxicity, but other common signs of this problem include fatigue, lethargy, headache, poor skin condition, acne, spots or pimples, bad breath, dark urine, pre-menstrual syndrome and cellulite.

In order to understand how toxicity in the body comes about, we must first understand the systems designed to keep the body pollutant-free. Central to these processes is an organ called the liver.

The liver

The liver is the body's largest solid organ, weighing about 2-2½ kg (5 lbs) in an adult. The liver sits in the upper right-hand side of the abdomen and is the primary organ of detoxification in the body. Blood that comes from the digestive tract goes first to the liver (via a vessel known as the hepatic portal vein). This means that anything potentially harmful to the body that starts out in the gut is passed directly to the liver. One of the liver's chief jobs is to process potential toxins so that they can be removed harmlessly from the body. In this way, the liver acts as a buffer between the gut and the rest of the body.

The liver also takes blood from the general circulation via a vessel called the hepatic artery. In this way, the liver is also exposed to toxins from other sources, including those inhaled through the lungs (e.g. cigarette smoke and pollution) and absorbed through the skin (e.g. cosmetics and detergents). So, wherever a toxin has come from, the chances are the liver will have a crack at dealing with it.

So, what exactly are all these toxins that the body has to deal with every day? Some of the potential hazards lurking in the body that keep the liver busy include:

- **Food additives, including artificial colourings and preservatives**
- **Artificial sweeteners**
- **Herbicides and pesticides**
- **Airborne pollutants**
- **Heavy metals such as mercury (from amalgam fillings)**
- **Toxins derived from cigarette smoke**
- **Hormone-like molecules (often derived from plastics) which may contaminate our food and water supply**
- **Naturally occurring food toxins**
- **Incompletely digested food molecules**
- **Cleaning substances and detergents**
- **Cosmetics and personal hygiene products**

- **Toxins produced from gut organisms (e.g. yeast, parasites and undesirable bacteria)**
- **Prescription medication**
- **Alcohol**
- **Recreational drugs**
- **Caffeine**

Because the liver is exposed to so many different types of potentially toxic substances, it has some pretty resourceful ways of dealing with them. Let's take a closer look at the processes the liver uses to neutralize unwanted substances that may be present in the body.

Liver detoxification – a two-stage process

The way the liver deals with toxins involves a two-stage process known as Phase 1 and Phase 2 detoxification. The first phase of detoxification involves a system of enzymes called cytochrome P450. Through a variety of reactions, toxins are treated in a way that makes it easier for them to be attached to other molecules. The significance of this will be apparent later.

Phase 1 detoxification is a good thing, but it is not without hazards. During this phase, destructive molecules called free radicals can be generated, which have the potential for damaging the liver. It is important, therefore, to ensure that the liver has an adequate supply of substances called antioxidants. Antioxidants quench free radicals and are able to protect the body from their damaging effects. More about these antioxidants later.

It is also important to bear in mind that efficient Phase 1 detoxification depends to a degree on the supply of certain nutrients. If these nutrients are not present in adequate amounts, there is a very real risk that Phase 1 detoxification will stall, eventually leading to a toxic build-up in the body. The natural substances that participate in liver detoxification will be covered at the end of this chapter.

Once toxins have been through the chemical processes of Phase 1 detoxification, it's time for them to pass on to the Phase 2 reactions. Many of the end products of Phase 1 detoxification are married with one of four carrier molecules in a process known as 'conjugation'. The products of these reactions can then be eliminated from the body. Some of these pass out in the urine, while others get dumped into bile and eventually make their way out of the body in the stool. As with the Phase 1 pathways, Phase 2 detoxification is also dependent on the supply of certain natural substances.

If, for any reason, either Phase 1 or Phase 2 detoxification is faulty, then problems with toxicity may arise. Sometimes liver function is generally good but it just gets overwhelmed by the sheer weight of the toxic load on it. Later in this chapter we shall be exploring ways of supporting liver function and reducing the quantity of toxins the body is exposed to. But first, let's take a closer look at the relationship between toxicity and weight.

The link between toxicity and weight gain

Weight loss is usually a welcome side effect of any detox programme. This phenomenon might be related to one or more possible mechanisms:

1. Toxins cause fat to accumulate

Toxins have an affinity for fat. In fact, they like to lodge themselves in the fat that is contained within the fat cells around the body. As a rule, the body does not like to let the concentration of potentially harmful substances rise too high and will usually put into place mechanisms to guard against this. One way to reduce toxicity is to clear them more quickly. However, if this is not appropriate, or just doesn't work quickly enough, the body's only other option is to 'dilute' the toxins. As the toxins generally sit around in the fat cells, this means that one way for the body to accommodate them is to make the fat cells bigger.

2. Toxins cause fluid retention

Another way that toxins may be diluted in the body is when fluid accumulates. Fluid retention (swollen ankles, puffy hands and face) is indeed a common factor in food intolerance, which is itself a frequent underlying feature in toxicity.

3. Toxins block reactions that burn food for energy

Central to weight control are the reactions that burn food to generate energy. If these reactions occur swiftly and efficiently, fuel is burnt more quickly and there is less likelihood that fat will accumulate. It may be that toxins in the body have the capacity to interfere with the body's metabolic reactions, causing them to stall and thus causing weight to accumulate.

Is toxicity your problem?

The following questionnaire is designed to help you assess whether toxicity is a problem in you. Score each question as indicated, and then add up your total score.

Do you suffer from:

1. Bad breath
No –   0 points
Occasional or mild problems – 2 points
Frequent or severe problems – 4 points

2. Abdominal bloating
No –   0 points
Occasional or mild problems – 2 points
Frequent or severe problems – 4 points

3. Constipation
No -   0 points
Occasional or mild problems – 2 points
Frequent or severe problems – 4 points

4. Fatigue
No –   0 points
Occasional or mild problems – 1 points
Frequent or severe problems – 2 points

5. Intolerance to rich and/or fatty food
No –   0 points
Occasional or mild problems – 2 points
Frequent or severe problems – 4 points

6. Food sensitivities
No –   0 points
Occasional or mild problems – 2 points
Frequent or severe problems – 4 points

7. Sensitivities to perfumes, paint fumes, traffic fumes or detergents

No –   0 points
Occasional or mild problems – 2 points
Frequent or severe problems – 4 points

8. Headaches

No –   0 points
Occasional or mild problems – 1 points
Frequent or severe problems – 2 points

9. Acne or spots

No –   0 points
Occasional or mild problems – 3 points
Frequent or severe problems – 5 points

10. Do you suffer from cellulite?

No –   0 points
Occasional or mild problems – 3 points
Frequent or severe problems – 5 points

11. Do you suffer from gallstones or episodes of gallbladder inflammation?

No –   0 points
Yes –   4 points

12. Have you ever suffered from hepatitis?

No –   0 points
Yes –   4 points

13. Are you frequently exposed to industrial or agricultural chemicals, such as solvents, paint fumes, plant sprays and fertilizers?

No –   0 points
Yes –   4 points

14. How many caffeinated drinks do you have in a day?

None –   0 points
1-3 –   3 points
4 or more –   6 points

15. How many units of alcohol do you consume each day on average?

0-1 –   0 points
2-3 –   3 points
4 or more –   6 points

Interpreting your score

0 – 9:   body toxicity is very unlikely
10 – 19:   body toxicity should be considered as a possibility
20 – 29:   body toxicity is quite likely, and steps taken to reduce this
                may well be beneficial
30 and above: body toxicity is very likely, and steps taken to reduce this
                will almost certainly be beneficial

Optimizing the body's detoxification processes

While liver function may be somewhat sluggish from time to time, the good news is that it has an enormous capacity for regeneration. Cut two-thirds of the liver away and it will regrow in a matter of a few months. The liver has an enormous potential for self-healing, just as long as it's given the opportunity.

The cornerstone of a liver-friendly programme is a healthy diet. Certain foods demand more work from the liver than others. While fruits, vegetables, beans, pulses and grains tend not to tax the liver, foods such as meat and dairy products do. The more the diet is based on foods which support liver function, rather than stress it, the more likely it is that the system will be clear and toxin-free. The essentials of a liver-supporting diet are:

1. The diet should contain an abundance of fresh fruits and vegetables. Not only do these foods tend not to tax and stress the liver, they also contain an abundance of nutrients, such as vitamin C and carotenoids (e.g. beta-carotene), which can support liver function. Try and include as many organic foods in your diet as possible.

2. Foods containing a lot of fat and/or protein should be downplayed in the diet, as they require quite a lot of chemical processing in the liver. The main foods to avoid are fatty meats such as beef, lamb and duck, dairy products and unhealthy hydrogenated vegetable oils present in margarine and many processed foods.

3. Foods containing artificial additives, such as sweeteners, colourings, flavourings and preservatives, should be minimized in the diet.

4. Alcohol, well known for its ability to stress the liver should be moderated, and preferably completely eliminated, during the initial phase of any detoxification regime.

5. Caffeine should also be moderated in the diet as it stresses the liver.

6. Plenty of fluid helps detoxification. About 1½ litres (2½ pt) of fluid each day is right for most people. Most of this should come in the form of still, filtered or mineral water. Other acceptable beverages include herb and fruit teas and diluted freshly squeezed fruit and vegetables juices.

Laboratory tests for a sluggish liver

If your doctor takes a blood sample to assess your liver function, it will normally be analysed for the level of certain liver-related substances. Some of the most commonly assessed liver-function tests are:

Bilirubin – a breakdown product of red blood cells. Levels of this substance can rise if the liver is not processing bile efficiently or if there is something causing obstruction to bile flow, such as gallstones.

Albumin – is a protein made in the liver. Its main function is to hold fluid in the blood vessels, thereby restricting the amount of fluid that escapes into the body's tissues. Liver disease can lead to low levels of albumin in the bloodstream, predisposing the body to fluid retention.

Alkaline phosphatase (AP) – an enzyme found in bile. Levels of this substance tend to go up when there is obstruction of the flow of bile from the liver.

The transaminases (aminotransferases) – a group of enzymes which tend to go up in the bloodstream once liver cells are damaged. Conditions such as hepatitis and excessive alcohol consumption can tend to elevate the level of the transaminases.

While liver-function tests can give quite a good guide to a liver problem when there is something quite serious going on, they are not necessarily sensitive enough to pick up more subtle imbalances. What this means is that many individuals who have problems with liver toxicity have completely normal liver-function tests. Individuals with symptoms which suggest a liver that is not quite keeping pace often have something going on in the gut that is causing the liver to be stressed. Some very important factors in this respect are food sensitivity, yeast overgrowth, leakiness in the gut wall and chronic constipation.

Food sensitivity and liver toxicity

There is a theory that before food is absorbed into the bloodstream from the gut, it is first broken down into its smallest molecular constituents. However, this does not necessarily seem to be the case. It appears as though undigested food molecules can make their way through the gut wall and can then go on to give rise to adverse reactions in the body, such as fluid retention, fatigue, eczema and arthritis. These reactions are often referred to as 'food intolerance'.

Once food leaves the digestive tract, the first place it goes is to the liver. The liver is not really designed to cope with partially digested food so these larger than normal molecules can really pose enormous problems for it. If you suspect liver toxicity, you need to give at least a passing thought to food sensitivity as a potential underlying factor in this. (For more details about food sensitivity, what it is, how it comes about and, most importantly of all, what to do about it, see chapter 6, *Eliminate Your Allergies*).

Yeast overgrowth and liver toxicity

In the gut large numbers of healthy bacteria reside and they play a variety of roles in the body, including assisting in digestion, keeping unhealthy organisms at bay and ensuring that the lining of the gut remains healthy. The gut also contains the yeast organism candida albicans and, as long as there is not too much of this around, it is unlikely to give us any problems. However, under certain circumstances, candida can overgrow in the gut and this can lead to a number of symptoms, including abdominal bloating, wind, fatigue, sweet or starch cravings and thrush (vaginal yeast infection). Candida is known to produce a range of potential toxins that have the capacity to get into the system by breaching the gut wall.

And, as if this was not enough, candida can also impair digestion and contribute to leakiness in the gut wall (see below). If you tend to feel that toxicity in your system is a problem and you suffer from some of the symptoms typical of candida overgrowth, it may well help you if you take steps to combat yeast in your body. (For more details about this see chapter 7, *Break the Mould*).

Leakiness in the gut wall and liver toxicity

It's only 3 mm (⅛ in) thick, but the lining of the gut wall provides an incredibly important barrier between the contents of the gut and the rest of the body, including the liver. Normally, only very small molecules can be admitted into the system through the gut wall. As far as the liver is concerned, the smaller the molecules it has to deal with, the better. Should the gut wall become somewhat leaky, then the liver may be exposed to toxins and food particles it is ill-equipped to deal with. Leakiness in the gut wall can actually be assessed with a laboratory test. In this test, the subject drinks a fluid containing molecules in a range of sizes. The urine is then collected and analysed for these molecules. If large molecules are found in the urine, this suggests leakiness in the gut.

Leaky gut tests (called 'tests for intestinal permeability') are available via specialist laboratories. For details about getting one of these tests, see the 'Useful Information' section at the back of the book. It is important to remember that leakiness in the gut is itself usually related to other factors, such as food sensitivity and candida overgrowth, and so considering these factors is important. It is advisable to work with a practitioner who is skilled at diagnosing gut and liver imbalance to help you pinpoint the underlying nature of your symptoms.

Constipation and liver toxicity

One of the main functions of the large bowel is to eliminate waste material from the gut. Sometimes bowel function is sluggish, leading to a problem with constipation.

There is no universally accepted definition of this term, but generally it is taken to mean either infrequent bowel motions, difficulty in passing stools or the incomplete passage of stools. Either way, constipation is not good for us. In the long term it may lead to problems such as diverticular disease (the development of small out-pocketings in the lining of the large bowel) and haemorrhoids (piles). However, as an everyday problem, constipation increases the likelihood that toxins in the waste material within the large bowel will be reabsorbed into the system, giving the liver more work to do.

Overcoming any degree of constipation is therefore important if the liver is to be kept as toxin-free as possible. The major underlying factors in constipation are:

1. Lack of fibre in the diet

Fibre in the diet is essential to give the bowel wall something to grip onto. A diet low in fibre and high in refined foods will almost certainly hamper the passage of waste material along the colon.

2. Lack of fluid

Just as important as fibre in healthy bowel function is fluid. If fluid intake into the body is low, the body will absorb as much of the water from the colon as possible. This can cause the faeces to become dry and difficult to pass.

3. Lack of exercise

Exercise can help stimulate the movement of matter along the large intestine, probably due to the mechanical action of the abdominal muscles and the diaphragm pushing against the bowel during exercise. A lack of exercise can therefore be a factor in constipation.

5. Pregnancy

Constipation is a common side effect of pregnancy. This can be explained, at least in part, by the presence of an enlarged womb pressing against the lower end of the large bowel.

6. Thyroid disease

The thyroid gland in the neck governs the body's metabolism. Should the thyroid become under-active, all of the body's major systems will slow down, including large bowel function. A common symptom of an underactive thyroid is therefore constipation.(For more details about thyroid disease, see chapter 4, *Keep up the Heat.*)

7. A tumour in the colon

A tumour of the large bowel can cause constipation. Often, the constipation will alternate with diarrhoea. Sometimes there may be blood in the bowel motion. Anyone over the age of 40 years who has had persistent changes in bowel habit should have this investigated by a doctor.

8. Drug therapy

Certain medications can cause constipation as a side effect. These include antacids, painkillers based on codeine and iron.

Combating constipation

Anyone who is prone to constipation may be tempted to use laxatives such as sennakot to relieve this. While these may temporarily relieve a constipation problem, many people find that they can become reliant on laxatives for their bowel function. Part of this is because laxatives may stimulate the gut abnormally, causing the gut to lose its ability to function properly. Also, laxatives often contain agents that irritate the lining of the gut, which is not good for general digestive health. As much as possible, any problems with constipation should be relieved naturally and the use of laxatives, especially in the long term, should be avoided.

1. Increase your intake of fibre

One essential ingredient for healthy bowel function is fibre. High-fibre breakfast cereals based on wheat bran are often advised for people suffering from constipation. However, the fibre in these cereals is quite hard and scratchy and may actually irritate the delicate lining of the gut. The fibre found in oats, fresh fruits and vegetables is generally much kinder to the gut and you should increase your consumption of these foods to relieve constipation. Aim at eating at least five servings of fruit or vegetables each day.

2. Use natural bulking agents

An effective way to increase your fibre intake is to add a natural bulking agent to your diet. These can really help to improve bowel regularity. Take one or two dessert spoonfuls of either psyllium husks or linseeds with some water each day.

3. Drink more water

Apart from fibre, the other essential ingredient for bowel regularity is fluid. However, some alcohol and drinks that contain alcohol can dehydrate the body and therefore worsen constipation. The best form of fluid for bowel health is water. Drink 1½–2 litres (2½–3 pt) of still water each day.

4. Take exercise

Exercise can help relieve constipation. Aim to take 30 minutes-worth of aerobic exercise (e.g. brisk walking, light jogging, cycling, rowing, aerobics, aqua-aerobics) at least three or four times a week.

5. Always respond to the call of nature

In the long term, failing to respond to the urge to open your bowels may cause a suppression of the process that is essential for defecation to take place.

Other detoxifying methods

As well as the methods outlined above, there are also some other methods that promote detoxification of the body. These are:

Fasting

Sometimes a good way to give the detoxification system a shove in the right direction is to fast. For many, fasting conjures up images of endless days subsisting on nothing but plain water. Actually, it doesn't have to be this way. There are variations of the water-only fast that may have tremendous benefit in terms of giving the body a decent detox in just a few days. Here's a good example of just such a fast:

The one week rice and vegetable fast

The concept for this fast is simple. Eat nothing but brown rice and raw and steamed vegetables for one week. The only fluid to be drunk is still mineral or filtered water, additive-free herb teas and freshly prepared vegetable juices. The benefits of this fast are that it does not encourage yeast overgrowth, is unlikely to include foods to which there may be a sensitivity (e.g. wheat, dairy), excludes foods and drinks that tend to stress the liver (meat, dairy, processed foods) but is nonetheless quite sustaining. If possible, the rice and vegetables should be organic, but this is not critical. If the food is not organic, make sure you give it a good, thorough washing before eating or cooking.

One of the great things about this fast is that because you can eat as much rice and vegetables as you like, there really is no need to be hungry. Bored yes, hungry no. Mind you, with the tremendous variety of vegetables now available to us, boredom does not to need not be a factor, either.

Once you come off this modified fast, it is probably not a good idea to go straight back to the diet you had previously. A better idea is to introduce food gently back into the diet. Perhaps some fish and fruit for the first few days, followed by a little meat if you eat this. Gradual reintroduction of foods allows your liver to become accustomed to a more varied and challenging diet over time.

A word of caution

During the initial stages of any detoxifying regime, it is not uncommon for individuals to feel worse, rather than better. The theory is that once the body has the opportunity, it may throw off toxins that may have been building up for a long time. Such a large outpouring of toxins from the body's cells can be too much for the liver, and the spill-over may give rise to symptoms such as headache, lethargy, achiness and mild flu-like symptoms. Detoxification reactions of this nature normally only last a few days but, if the system is very toxic or if the liver function is very compromised, symptoms may persist for two weeks or more. To help minimize the adverse effects of a fast or cleansing regime, it is important to ensure that plenty of fluids are taken to help flush toxins out through the urine, together with liver-supporting nutrients. These nutrients are listed in the section on supplements at the end of this chapter.

Saunas and steam baths

One way the body can eliminate toxins is through sweating. This is certainly not the main way that the body rids itself of toxins, but it's not insignificant. Because saunas and steam baths encourage sweating, they can be a useful adjunct to any detoxification programme, 20–30 minutes of body sweating, two or three times a week, can help keep the system clean.

Skin brushing

Toxins tend to accumulate in the fat cells and the lymphatic system of the body. The lymphatic system is made up of a network of vessels, along which are stationed collections of immune cells called lymph nodes. The lymphatic vessels take tissue debris and many of the end products of cell metabolism and shunt these to the lymph nodes, where immune cells process and deactivate them before they are dumped into the body's circulation. In this way, the lymphatic system functions as a sort of sewage disposal system. It is thought that lymph fluid can become somewhat sluggish, causing toxins to accumulate. Incidentally, accumulation of toxins in the lymph system and fat cells at the back of the thighs is probably a major factor in the development of cellulite.

Skin brushing can be used to help shift lymph fluid and the toxins contained within it, and can be a useful technique in combating cellulite and promoting detoxification. Skin brushes made of natural fibre can be found in health food stores. Ideally, skin brushing should be performed on dry skin for about five minutes, twice a day. The brush should be used quite vigorously on the legs and arms, and the direction of brushing should always be towards the heart. If cellulite is a problem, particular attention should be given to the back of the legs.

Lymphatic massage

Another way lymph fluid can be coaxed into a more fluid state is through massage. Aromatherapy, sports, and beauty-based massages are unlikely to do the trick here. What is needed is a practitioner who has been trained in what is known as manual lymphatic drainage (MLD). (For details about how to go about finding a MLD practitioner, see the 'Useful Information' section at the back of the book.)

Colonic irrigation

Colonic irrigationists generally believe that the large bowel can harbour undigested food matter and other nasties that have accumulated over many years and that these may compromise health by fouling up the system. Clearing out this debris using warm water, and sometimes natural agents, is claimed to help reduce toxicity in the body and improve health. This form of natural therapy does tend to polarize people somewhat. Some hate it and find the whole idea utterly repulsive; others love it and claim it is a great way to clear out old toxins and rejuvenate the body. I have seen many individuals whose health has improved through colonic irrigation, particularly those who have bowel-related symptoms such as chronic constipation, flatulence, erratic bowel habit or haemorrhoids (piles).

Supporting the liver with supplements

Natural medicine has thrown up an array of agents that may help support liver function and the process of detoxification. Some of the more important nutrients include:

Milk thistle – milk thistle is a herb that's use as a natural remedy can be traced back more than 2,000 years. The herb contains a complex of bioflavonoid molecules, known collectively as silymarin, which appear to have the ability to protect the liver cells by reducing the take-up and enhancing the removal of harmful toxins (1,2). Silymarin also has powerful antioxidant activity (3) and can help in the regeneration of injured liver cells (4).

Inositol – this nutrient, which is generally classified as part of the B vitamin complex, helps in the breakdown and utilisation of fat and cholesterol and can help to reduce fatty build-up in the liver.

Choline – similar in action to inositol, this nutrient helps reduce fatty build-up in the liver and also helps the liver detoxify the by-products of protein metabolism.

Biotin – generally regarded as one of the B-complex vitamins, biotin participates in fat metabolism and can therefore help in the processing of fat in the liver.

Methionine – this amino acid is essential to good liver function and also helps the liver detoxify the by-products of protein metabolism.

Taurine – this is another important amino acid for the liver and can help reduce fatty build-up here.

Lipase – this a fat-digesting enzyme. Lipase helps reduce the fatty load on the liver and may help to keep the liver cells free from fat.

Alpha lipoic acid – this nutrient is a powerful antioxidant and has the power to protect the liver from free radical damage. It also participates in the recycling and regeneration of other liver-protecting antioxidants.

Green tea extract – is a rich source of substances called polyphenols, which have potent antioxidant activity. Like alpha lipoic acid, they can also participate in maintaining the activity of other liver protective substances.

Suggested supplement:

Hepranol – is a combination supplement containing a range of liver-supporting and detoxifying ingredients, such as milk thistle, choline, inositol, lipase, methionine, taurine, alpha lipoic acid and green tea extract. Long-term supplementation with Hepranol may assist liver function and reduce body toxicity. The normal recommended dose is one capsule, twice a day with food.

Availability

For details of how to obtain Hepranol see the 'Useful Information' section at the back of the book under the name *VitaTech*.

Case Study

Fiona D is a 31-year-old actress

> *I think my problems started just four or five years ago. I was never huge, but did have the propensity to fluctuate between nine and ten stones. I felt great at nine, and lousy at ten. Increasingly, I was finding it difficult to*

keep my weight under control. I had given up trying to get down to nine stones, and settled for nine and a half instead.

Apart from struggling with my weight, I had developed a new bunch of problems. Firstly, I found that I was starting to suffer from pimples around my jaw line. I was a little put out, to say the least. I had never had skin problems during adolescence and, as an actress, my appearance is very important to me. I would buy all sorts of creams and potions, but the skin problem persisted. I saw a dermatologist who suggested antibiotics, but I just couldn't bring myself to take them. Almost as bad as the spots was the cellulite. For years I would hear some of my friends moaning about it, but I never had a problem. Gradually, I found that the skin on my thighs and buttocks was looking orange-peely, and I was not happy!

One day, I was reading about detoxification in a women's magazine. It occurred to me that the spots, cellulite and the weight thing could all be explained by toxins. I was not working at the time and so I decided to give my body a spring clean. I must admit, I was not leading the healthiest lifestyle, anyway and thought this might do me good. I was prone to eating junk, especially when I was working, and I was quite into coffee and red wine. I thought it would do me good to give my body a break.

The detox programme in the magazine seemed a bit extreme to me so I did my own version of it. I cut out dairy products, meat and processed foods. I took out all grains, too, other than rice. For a month I basically lived on fish, fruit, veg and rice. If I went out to eat, I'd just have fish and veg. I stopped the coffee (hard) and wine (nightmare!) and just drank water. Some days I would get through two litres or more. At first the water was boring, but then I really got into it. Two more things I did was to skin brush and take a liver supplement. The article mentioned milk thistle, so I went to a health food stores and bought some.

I must admit, the first week on the plan was hard. I think I really missed the coffee. I had a whacking headache for the first three days but, thankfully, this went on the fourth day and never came back. My skin worsened, but the article said this often happens. Anyway, I stuck it out *and by the end of the week I was feeling much better. I think I must have lost three or four pounds that week (I wasn't weighing myself), and definitely had a boost in energy. I'm sure my thinking was clearer. The diet and the skin brushing were helping my cellulite and my skin was beginning to clear.*

Three weeks into the regime, I felt on top of the world. I felt so much slimmer and my friends started to notice just how much healthier I was looking. They kept asking me if I was on a diet. I took great pride in telling them that, no, I was doing a 'detox'. My complexion was looking fantastic and my cellulite had all but disappeared. I was thrilled. I started to relax things a little after the month was up. The wine crept back in, but I never felt the need to put coffee back in my diet. Mind you, I still drink masses of water and the skin brushing has become part of my regime.

I learnt a lot going through the detox plan. Somehow, I feel much more in control of my health. Even now, if I have a heavy weekend or something, I'll just go on a nice, clean diet for a week, and I'll be back to normal. I really do feel as though I've got off some sort of slippery slope.

Summary

- Toxicity is an important cause of weight gain and other health issues.

- Toxins can come from the outside (e.g. pollutants, food toxins) or the inside (e.g. by-products of metabolism).

- The function of the liver is key to the elimination of potentially toxic substances.

- The liver neutralizes toxins using a two-stage process.

- A liver-supporting diet is one which includes easily digested food, such as fruit, vegetables and grains, and is low in liver-taxing foods, such as fatty foods, dairy products, processed foods, alcohol and caffeine.

- Toxicity can be related to other factors, such as food sensitivity, candida overgrowth, leakiness in the gut wall and constipation.

- Modified fasting can be a useful way to kick-start the detoxification process.

- Sauna, steam baths, skin brushing, lymph drainage massage and colonic irrigation may also help the detoxification process.

- Certain nutrients and herbs, including milk thistle, choline, inositol, green tea extract and alpha lipoic acid, can be very effective in improving liver function and reducing toxicity in the long term.

- For some individuals, detoxification can lead to significant weight loss and health rejuvenation.

CHAPTER 9

Breathe Away

If someone told you it was possible to lose weight without changing your diet or exercise regime, and without having to take any pills or potions, would you believe them? Probably not. However, what you will discover in this chapter is that it is possible to lose weight just by doing something that you already do – breathing. Now, while you may consider that breathing is something you do perfectly well without any tuition, there is good reason to believe that many of us fail to get adequate amounts of oxygen into our systems, and this can put a major brake on our metabolism. Oxygen is an essential ingredient in the reactions that take place to burn food and convert it to energy. Any shortfall in supply of this gas can stall any attempt to lose weight, and lead to significant problems with energy, too. Just practising a few simple breathing exercises each day can help to spark life into a flagging metabolism, and bring about weight loss and increased vitality.

The breath of life

While it may seem obvious that oxygen is absolutely essential to life, it is useful to understand what oxygen actually does in the body. Our need for oxygen cannot be overstated. The human body can survive a few weeks without food, and a few days without water, but it can't do without oxygen for more than a few minutes. Conditions such as heart attacks and strokes are caused by parts of the body becoming starved of oxygen due to an interruption in blood supply. Individuals who suffer from chronic lung diseases, such as chronic bronchitis and emphysema are usually prone to breathlessness, fatigue and a reduced capacity for exercise and activity. In short, oxygen is of prime importance to life and health.

So, what is the link between oxygen and weight? Can it really be that oxygen not only keeps us alive, but also slims us down, too? The answers to these questions is yes, and the reason for this phenomenon lies in the fact that the reactions which burn food and fuel stores require oxygen to function efficiently and completely. Take a look at this equation:

$$\text{Food + oxygen} \longrightarrow \text{energy (and weight loss)}$$

Many weight loss approaches focus intimately on getting the food part of this equation right. Very few, if any, consider the other major component, oxygen. The fact is, without adequate supplies of oxygen, it is simply not possible for the body to burn food effectively. You may remember the body furnace analogy in chapter 2, where the food we eat is represented by the fuel in the furnace, and the body's metabolism is represented by how well the fire is burning. Essentially, one of the main themes of this chapter is that when we decrease our fuel supply, the speed that the fuel burns (our metabolism) decreases, too. Well, another way to put a fire out is to starve it of oxygen. It's easy to see just how essential efficient breathing is in the maintenance of a healthy metabolism. Increasing the amount of oxygen delivered to our body's cells really can help us lose weight and regain vitality.

Are you breathing right?

Breathing really is one of those things that most of us assume we all do perfectly well. However, we know that the efficiency of basic systems in the body can vary enormously between individuals. While some people have cast-iron digestions and are able to break down and absorb any food without ill-effect, others may not be so lucky and so, as a result, run into problems with nutrient deficiency and food sensitivity. While certain individuals may have strong immune systems and get through the year without so much as a sniffle, others may be floored by just about any bug that happens to be lurking in their immediate environment. The same is true of breathing. Some people undoubtedly get all the oxygen they need for optimum health through their complete and efficient breathing habits, while others just don't quite cut it in this department, with potentially serious consequences for their weight and general vitality.

The act of breathing

Breathing fulfils two main functions in the body. As we know, all the cells in the body require oxygen to function, and the act of breathing allows this gas to be absorbed from the air into the bloodstream. But more about that later. While the cells use oxygen, they also generate a waste product called carbon dioxide. The other function of breathing is to allow the body to rid itself of this unwanted gas. The process of oxygen absorption and carbon dioxide elimination by the body is sometimes referred to as 'gas exchange'.

The structure and function of the lungs

Oxygen is taken into the body from the air via the lungs. Air, which is inhaled through the nose and/or mouth, first travels down the windpipe (trachea) to enter two tubes called the bronchi, each of which takes the air into each lung. The bronchi divide again and again, forming a branching network of tubes that get ever smaller in size as they approach the outer reaches of the lung tissue. Finally, these tubes end in the form of tiny sacs called alveoli. It is in the alveoli that all the action takes place. Surrounding the alveoli is an intimate network of tiny blood vessels known as capillaries. Air can pass back and forth between the alveoli and the blood in the capillaries, and this allows the lungs to perform their function of gas exchange.

When oxygen is breathed into the lungs, some of it will transfer across the wall of the alveoli into the blood contained in the capillaries. This blood (known as oxygenated blood) eventually travels to the heart in a vessel called the pulmonary vein. The heart then pumps this blood to the body's tissues, where the oxygen is used and swapped for carbon dioxide. This blood (known as deoxygenated blood) travels back to the heart, so that it can pump it once again to the lungs. In the lungs, the carbon dioxide leaves the bloodstream and enters the alveoli, after which it can be removed from the body as the lungs breathe out. On the in-breath, more oxygen is absorbed into the bloodstream from the air, and this then travels to the heart to be pumped to the rest of the body. And so this cycle repeats.

The act of breathing and the process of gas exchange depend on the mechanics that get air in and out of the lungs. Inspiration (breathing in) and expiration (breathing out) is controlled by muscular contractions in and around the chest. This is how breathing actually takes place. The chest cavity is essentially made up of the spine at the back, the sternum or breastbone at the front and ribs on either side which connect the two. After breathing out, the curved ribs hang down somewhat, rather like bucket handles (see diagram 2, below). Between the ribs are muscles (called intercostal muscles) which contract during inspiration. The effect of the intercostal muscle contraction is to draw the ribs up, increasing the size of the chest, which in turn causes air to be drawn into the lungs (inspiration).

Apart from the intercostal muscles there are other muscles involved in the act of breathing, the most important of which is the diaphragm. The diaphragm is a dome-shaped, thin, muscular sheet that lines the base of the chest and separates it from the abdomen. During inspiration, the diaphragm contracts and flattens, and this causes air to be drawn into the lungs.

Broadly speaking, individuals can be classified as 'chest breathers' or 'diaphragmatic (belly) breathers'. Chest breathers tend to breathe in an out using mainly their intercostal muscles. The breaths tend to be shallow and often relatively short. In chest breathing, air is drawn into the smaller upper parts of the lungs, but may never make it into the lower reaches of the lung where much of gas exchange

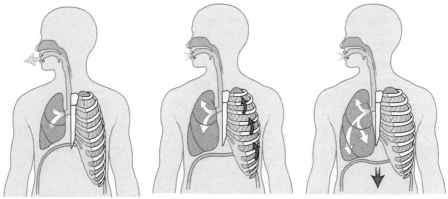

1. Exhalation   **2. Chest inhalation**   **3. Belly inhalation**

takes place. It is worth noting that in Eastern medicine, this type of breathing is viewed as inefficient and incomplete.

Belly breathing, on the other hand, is viewed as both healthy and important to well-being. Here, instead of the intercostal muscles doing the work, it is the diaphragm that contracts to draw air into the lungs. In diaphragmatic breathing, inspired air can make its way into the expansive lung tissue at the base of the chest.

Belly breathing goes a long way towards optimizing the process of oxygen absorption and carbon dioxide removal.

Are you a belly or chest breather?

This simple exercise will enable you to get a good idea of whether you are predominantly a chest breather or belly breather:

Put your left hand in the middle or your chest with your right hand over your navel. Breathe normally. Look at your hands and take a note of which hand moves more when you breathe. If your left hand is moving more than your right, it is a sign that you are a chest breather. If your right is moving more than your left, it is likely that you're breathing is essentially diaphragmatic in nature.

Is inefficient breathing your problem?

The following questionnaire is designed to help you assess the efficiency of your breathing. Score each question as indicated, and then add up your total score.

1. Having done the exercise above, do you rate yourself as a:
chest breather?–   8 points
belly breather? –   0 points
somewhere in between? – 4 points

2. Can walking up just one or two flights of stairs make you very breathless?
never –   0 points
sometimes –   2 point
often or always –   4 points

3. You are sometimes aware of the need to take a big breath of air at rest?
never –   0 points
sometimes –   2 points
often –   4 points

4. Do you consider yourself as a:
generally relaxed individual who is not prone to bouts of anxiety
or stress? –   0 points
highly strung and anxious individual who quite often feels anxious or
stressed out –   4 points
somewhere in between –   2 points

5. Count the number of breaths you take in a minute at rest (no sooner than an hour after any form of exercise). Do this three times during the day and average the result. Is the number of breaths you take in a minute:
5 – 9? –   0 points
between 10–15? –   3 points
16 or more? –   6 points

Interpreting your score
0 – 8:   your answers suggest that you have good breathing habits, and that poor breathing is unlikely to be an issue in your weight or health problems

10 – 14:   your answers suggest that your breathing habits may benefit from the breathing exercises outlined in this chapter

16 and above: your answers suggest that your breathing pattern is not healthy and that you would almost certainly benefit from practising the breathing techniques outlined in this chapter on a regular basis

Belly breathing exercise

If you have identified yourself as a bit of a chest breather, it will help you to learn the art of proper belly breathing. Even if you think you breathe mainly from the diaphragm, the following exercise is likely to help you make your breathing even more complete and efficient.

Breathe gently in and out through your nose. Breathe out all the air from your lungs, pause briefly, and begin to breathe in again. Concentrate on taking long, smooth, unhurried breaths.

As you breathe in, push your belly out. This will ensure you are filling the whole of your lungs with air. When your lungs feel comfortably full of air, pause briefly again and then breathe out slowly and evenly through your nose. Repeat this cycle, always making sure that your belly is moving in and out as you breathe.

If you're not used to deep breathing exercises, and particularly if you tend to chest breathe, you might be very pleasantly surprised at just how quick and effective this is for reviving your energy and clearing your head. Just ten breaths are all that you normally need to take for the benefits of deep breathing to be felt. Remember, if more oxygen is generating more energy, it is likely that more fuel is being burnt.

Although belly breathing takes some conscious effort to begin with, practise certainly does make perfect. In time you may well find that deep, diaphragmatic breathing comes as second nature to you.

I generally recommend that individuals who are learning belly breathing start with ten good breaths, three times a day. In most cases this really does seem to be enough to get things started. Within a couple of weeks, and often within just a few days, individuals normally feel that they've got the hang of diaphragmatic breathing, and may be extending their ten breaths to twenty or more at a time without even thinking about it. From time to time, it's a good idea to do the hand test to see whether or not you tend to belly or chest breathe at rest. You may be surprised to find that your old chest breathing habits give way to healthier and invigorating belly breathing in time.

More breathing exercises

There are a couple of exercises based on belly breathing I like myself and often teach to clients. Pauses between inhalation and expiration maximize the effect.

Breathing in threes

Take a good long belly breath and count 'one thousand, two thousand' and so on in your head while you do this. Once you have inhaled fully, hold your breath for the same number of counts as it took you to inhale, and then exhale completely over the same number of counts again. For instance, if you inhale to the count of six, hold your breath for six counts, exhale for six counts and then repeat this cycle. I generally recommend ten to fifteen cycles, repeated three times a day.

To begin with, you may need to adjust your count until you find a length of time you are comfortable with. If you go too slowly to begin with, you may find that you start to run out of breath and are unable to complete the exercise. If your breaths are too quick, you are unlikely to get the maximum benefit from them.

Breathing in fours

Breathing in fours is very similar to breathing in threes. The only difference is that after exhalation, the breath is held for the same count as the other components of the cycle. As an example, breathe in over six counts, hold for six counts, breathe out for six counts, hold for six counts and repeat. Breathing in fours is a little more challenging than breathing in threes and is something to progress to once you're comfortable with the easier exercise. I recommend ten to fifteen cycles, repeated three times a day, once you're proficient.

Case Study

Jane P is a 29-year-old marketing manager

> *I've had a problem with my weight since I was a teenager. At 16 years of age I was 5'4" and weighed eleven stones. By the time I was 23, I was weighing about 13½ stone. I would usually be watching my diet, and tended to yo-yo a bit over the years. My energy wasn't great either. I would tend to go to the gym in fits and starts, but it was always a bit of an effort to go.*

> *About eighteen months ago I started doing yoga. During the first session we spent most of the time practising proper breathing. Almost immediately, I felt like I had more energy and my mind started to buzz. I resolved, if nothing else, to keep the breathing exercises going, even if I couldn't manage the yoga twice a week. So, three times a day, I would stop to take ten long deep breaths. It didn't matter where I was. Pretty much whatever I was doing, I would just do them. Sitting in the car, standing in the shower, I remember doing them in a restaurant when my boyfriend had got up to go to the loo.*

> *Quite unexpectedly I noticed that I was beginning to lose weight. I lost four pounds in weight the week after I started the yoga classes. Initially, I did not make the connection between the weight loss and the breathing. I thought it was just one of those things. I mentioned it to my yoga instructor and she said she knew loads of people who have lost weight using breathing exercises. I ended up losing seven pounds in the first month alone.*

As it turned out, the yoga did fall by the wayside, but I felt so good about the breathing I just kept going. Very gradually I continued to lose weight, and eventually got down to about nine stones, which is a comfortable weight for me. Now I have bags more energy than I used to have. I really had no idea that something as simple as a few breathing exercises could make such a profound difference to my health.

Summary

- Oxygen is an essential ingredient in the reactions that convert food into energy.

- Insufficient oxygen or inefficient breathing technique may stall the metabolism and lead to problems with weight gain and/or low energy.

- Inefficient breathers tend to breathe into the upper chest, while efficient breathers tend to breathe into the lower reaches of the lungs using the diaphragm.

- Learning diaphragmatic or belly breathing is the first step in developing healthy breathing habits.

- Once belly breathing is mastered, moving on to more ambitious exercises such as breathing in threes and breathing in fours can help maximize the effect.

- Good breathing habits can be an effective way to lose weight and restore vitality.

10

Move It

It won't come as any surprise that a book that purports to take a truly holistic approach to the subjects of weight loss and health should include a chapter about exercise. Mind you, despite the fact that I've always had a keen interest in sport and exercise, take exercise most days and know the basics of sports physiology, I'm certainly no expert. For this reason I enlisted Chris Williams, an exercise specialist, to help me write this chapter. During our research I learnt that, contrary to popular opinion, relatively short periods of quite strenuous activity can be very effective for losing weight. More revelations came when I discovered that strength training is a great way to lose weight, too.

These ideas fly a little in the face of conventional exercise-related wisdom but they are actually backed up by sound physiological principles. A little later, we'll be discussing the rationale of this new thinking. First, though, we have to understand how the body is fuelled during exercise.

Food for sport

The body derives its energy during exercise from three main fuel stores. The immediate fuel the body uses to generate energy is sugar in the blood. However, the total amount of sugar in the blood only provides a very small energy reservoir, so the level of blood sugar must be continually topped-up during exercise. The body keeps a large fuel store for this purpose in the form of a substance called glycogen, which is similar in structure to starch. Glycogen is stored in the muscles and the liver and is quite readily converted into sugar, which can then be burnt for energy. The third energy store in the body is fat. Much more energy can be stored as fat in the body than glycogen, but the body finds it harder to convert this form of fuel into energy.

Imagine that fuel sources used to fuel exercise are like money. We can think of sugar in the bloodstream as the money in our pocket or purse: easy to get hold of, but in relatively short supply. Glycogen we can think of as our current account: necessary in order to keep the money in our purse or pocket topped up, but a bit harder to get hold of. Finally, fat can be thought of as a sort of deposit account: where the bulk of our money is kept but to which our access is more limited.

Also, it is worth bearing in mind that although fat may make up the predominant fuel source during less strenuous exercise, this generally doesn't happen for a good fifteen minutes or so after exercise begins. It takes this long for fat to be burnt in appreciable quantities. This means that at whatever intensity you are exercising, relatively small amounts of fat will be burnt until you have been exercising for quite a considerable amount of time.

Long and slow – the conventional approach to weight loss

If you've followed the story so far, then you'll understand why conventional wisdom has been that in order to lose weight through exercise it's important to engage in relatively prolonged periods of not too strenuous exercise. Because of this thinking, gyms and sports clubs are usually awash with individuals attempting to lose weight by doing exercise sessions made up of 15 minutes on the jogging machine followed by 15 minutes on a bike followed by 10 minutes on the step machine. However, it now appears that the 'long and slow' philosophy for weight loss through exercise might be a little off track.

A new way of looking at weight loss through exercise

Let's imagine you decide you're going to run 5 km (3 miles) outside or on a treadmill. One way to complete the distance would be to walk at, say, a 5 km/hr (3 miles/hr) pace. So, you'll cover the 5 km (3 miles) in an hour and, depending on factors such as your size, metabolism and fitness level, you'll expend about 260 calories doing this. About half of those calories will come from fat, the rest will come from carbohydrate stores. So, at a slow pace, you'll burn about 130 fat calories covering 5 km (3 miles).

Now, imagine you've decided you're going to get through the 5 km (3 miles) a bit more quickly. Imagine you set out to cover the 5 km (3 miles) in 40 minutes (7½ km/hr [4½ miles/hr]). The fuel consumption of the body varies according to speed. At faster speeds the body tends to use more fuel. This is similar to the effect you see when driving a car. If you drive very quickly, the amounts of fuel you use over a given distance is greater than when you drive at a more moderate speed, despite the fact that you're driving for a shorter period of time. At 7½ km/hr (4½ miles/hr), you'll burn about 400 calories covering 5 km (3 miles). The percentage of these calories supplied by fat will be less than before (about 40%) because the activity is more strenuous, but this still adds up to 160 calories of fat. In other words, if we step up the pace a little, we can burn more calories and, most importantly, more fat calories, and it takes less time, too!

Does this mean that low intensity exercise is no good?

Not at all. If you don't take any real exercise at the moment, then any intensity of exercise is likely to benefit you from a weight loss and health-related benefit point of view. However, the bottom line is this: if you can comfortably and safely exercise at a higher intensity, then it's probably going to pay you to do this. Later on in the chapter we'll be covering some exercise and activity programmes, the least strenuous of which is based on walking. If you haven't taken exercise for a while, then this would be an ideal place to start. Before we look at the programmes, though, we should examine the issue of how much exercise is the optimum for achieving weight loss and improved fitness.

How much exercise?

To get a real weight-loss and health-related benefit, you're probably going to need to set aside enough time to take half an hour's-worth of exercise about four times a week. Five times is better, but three will do. These figures are only guides. If you can only grab twenty minutes of exercise twice a week, then that's considerably better than none at all. So, do whatever you can manage and be satisfied with what you have achieved. If you can manage to do a little more exercise the next week, fine. If you can't, then that's fine, too.

As we have already discussed earlier, the intensity of the exercise you take does have an affect on how much fat you burn and how much weight you lose. Since the 1960s, the heart rate has been used as a measure of the intensity of exercise. It has been established that an exercise effort of between 60-80% maximum heart rate (MHR) is sufficient to gain fitness and health benefits. The MHR is the rate at which the heart rate peaks with maximum effort. The MHR or individual can be estimated using the following formula:

Maximum Heart Rate = 220 – age

The maximum heart rate for a 40-year-old is therefore 180. This equates to a target heart rate of between 108 and 144.

To find out whether you are exercising to the correct intensity, stop exercising for a moment to take your pulse. The pulse can be felt on the inside of your wrist close to the base of your thumb. Count the number of beats you feel in 15 seconds. Using the example above for a 40-year-old, the number of beats in 15 seconds should be between 27 and 36.

A more high-tech approach to this would be to invest in something called a heart-rate monitor. Essentially, this consists of a band worn around the chest and a watch. The band contains a heart beat sensing device, which is then beamed to the watch for display. There are some very fancy heart-rate monitors available that you probably don't need. The basic models are generally inexpensive and can be bought in good sports stores.

Now, if calculating your ideal heart-rate range and taking your pulse or buying a heart rate monitor all seems like too much of an effort, and I do sympathize with you if that's the case, then you might want to take a low-tech approach. Generally, if you are doing any aerobic activity such as brisk walking, jogging, cycling and rowing, you should aim to be so breathless that you can just about snatch a conversation (more information on aerobic exercises can be found later in this chapter). This way, you'll be working hard enough to be getting real benefit at a pace you can sustain.

Some general guidelines about exercise

If you haven't exercised for a while, and even if you have, it may be worthwhile taking note of the following general points.

1. Get checked out

If you suffer from a significant illness, such as heart disease, high blood pressure or an arthritic condition, it is a good idea to check with your doctor to see if you are fit enough to exercise.

2. Get in gear

You might need to invest in some suitable exercise clothing. I would suggest that the only piece of clothing you really need is a good pair of running shoes or cross trainers. These will help ensure that you do not jar your body during exercise, reducing the risk muscle and joint injury.

3. Keep hydrated

Get into the habit of drinking plenty of water on a daily basis. Having water on board before you exercise is known to enhance performance. Keeping a small bottle of water with you when you exercise and taking sips from this is a good idea too.

4. Get planning

If you have a busy life, don't expect exercise slots to just pop up in your diary. Part of the secret to getting more exercise into your life is to schedule activity sessions in advance. Chris Williams tells his clients to put exercise sessions in their diaries just as they would schedule meetings, or lunches. I think this is a goood idea.

5. Warm up

Any exercise session is best preceded by a 5-minute warm-up. Taking some very gentle exercise to begin with prepares the body for the more strenuous activity ahead. During a warm-up, you will get the heart rate up a bit, increase muscle temperature, activate cooling mechanisms in the body and mobilise the joints. Brisk walking or light jogging is an ideal way to warm up. Straight after the warm-up, take a few minutes to stretch (see opposite).

6. Cool down

Just as the body should be started up slowly, it should be turned down slowly, too. What this means is that after each session it's a good idea to go through a period of cooling down. One of the main benefits of cooling down is that it can help in the elimination of waste products from the muscles, which reduces the risk of soreness setting in a day or two later. So, if you started your session with five minutes of brisk walking or light jogging, repeat these exercises at the end of the session. After the cool down, stretch again.

7. Listen to your body

If at any point during exercise you feel faint, dizzy, develop chest pain, have unusual difficulty breathing or experience severe muscular or joint discomfort, stop immediately. If the symptoms persist, seek medical attention. Individuals with a history of high blood pressure or heart disease should be especially suspicious of symptoms such as unusual shortness of breath or chest pain.

Stretch it out

Stretching needs to form an integral part of any exercise programme as it encourages muscle and joint flexibility. This is important, because even if you are fit and strong, if you lose flexibility, you lose function. Between the ages of 20 and 70, we can expect to lose about 40% of our flexibility. This has an enormous impact on our ability to do whatever we want to do in our lives, whether it's gardening, dancing, golf, marathon running or just getting out of a bed or a chair without the need of assistance.

The following stretch routine ideally should be performed every day, and before and after you take exercise. Stretching is best performed after a short warm-up, as warm muscles are more pliable and less prone to injury.

Each stretch should be performed in a slow, controlled manner. The muscle group being stretched should be taken to a point where it starts to offer some resistance. At this point a little more tension can be applied, but not so much that the muscle hurts. The stretch should be steady – no bouncing! Hold each stretch for a steady count of 20, but do remember to keep breathing throughout.

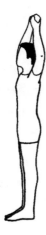

1. Overarm shoulder stretch

Clasp your hands together above your head with your elbows slightly bent. Slowly push your arms backward and hold. Keep looking forward and remember to keep your neck in a comfortable position at all times (avoid craning your head and neck forwards).

2. Underarm shoulder stretch

Clasp your hands behind your back, with your elbows slight bent. Slowly raise your arms and hold. Do not bend forward, and remember to keep your neck in a comfortable position throughout.

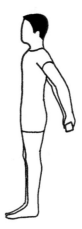

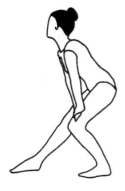

3. Hamstring stretch

Place your right foot one step in front of the left. Lean forward by bending at the waist, keeping your back straight and your head up. Support both of your hands on the top of your left thigh. Slowly drop your hips and buttocks backward and downward until you can feel mild tension in the back of the right thigh. Keep your right knee slightly bent throughout this exercise. Repeat this stretch on the other side.

4. Quadricep stretch

Facing a wall, support your body with your left arm by placing your hand against the wall. Lift your right leg up towards the back, until you can grasp and hold your right foot in your right hand. Slowly ease the heel of the foot toward the buttocks. Hold. Keep your left leg slightly bent throughout this exercise. Keep your knees together and keep your back straight. Repeat this stretch on the other side.

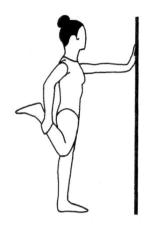

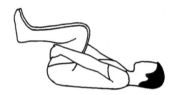

5. Back stretch

Lie on your back with your knees bent. Hold the back of your thighs. Slowly pull your knees towards your chest with your hands clasped behind your thighs. Hold and then relax.

Training programmes

Here is a guide to some of the exercise sessions you can incorporate into your life in order to lose weight and enhance your health. What Chris and I have tried to do here is give you very simple, low-tech programmes, which do not require you to go to a gym or invest in any fancy equipment. Now, if you want to do that, that is fine. However, our belief is that exercise should be easy and something you can do in your home or from your front door. The exercises suggestions that are given here are based on three principal activities:

1. **Walking**
2. **Jogging**
3. **A home circuit session based on both strength and aerobic activities**

Take a walk

I rate walking as an excellent form of exercise. You can undoubtedly burn fat calories doing it, and it's also cheap, convenient, recreational and needs no special equipment other than a decent pair of trainers. Now, if the idea of walking for exercise conjures up images for you of lone individuals in top-to-toe sports gear walking determinedly on treadmills, then you may do well to consider other options. You can don all the gear and join a swanky gym if you want, but there are plenty of other ways, too. Maybe you want to walk outside, in a local park, for instance. Perhaps you want to take a partner with you – a sort of walking buddy. Maybe the dog wants to come, too. The main thing here is that you should do whatever you enjoy the most. And maybe that will vary from day to day.

I remember I was in Malta a few years ago, training with my cousin at the national sports arena. Walking briskly around the outside of the running track were two Maltese ladies in their sixties, wearing everyday clothing apart from running shoes on their feet. They had started walking before I began my own training session (a six-mile run), and were still going after I'd finished. I was most impressed!

A little word of advice about the walking itself: in general, it is better to take quick steps rather than long strides. Longer steps are hard on the joints, especially the knees, and don't allow you to go any faster. Take steps just slightly longer than you would normally, landing on your heels and rolling through to your toes.

Although walking is predominantly a lower body exercise, there's no reason why you shouldn't get you upper body involved. Bend your elbows to 90 degrees, relax your shoulders and swing away as you go. This helps you to use more energy and give you a better overall workout at the same time.

As your fitness improves you may find that you are able to step up the pace without getting any more tired. From time to time, you might want to check how long it takes you to get round a set course. Sometimes it helps, especially during the initial stages of a new exercise regime, to get objective proof of your progress. A word of warning here, for goodness sake do not become a slave to the stopwatch. There can be a tendency for individuals who get into timing to get competitive with themselves, often looking to achieve faster and faster times. There will come a point, and this does happen to everyone (even world class athletes), where they just can't go any faster, and this may turn out to be a bit of a de-motivator. Besides, getting all fussed about times and speeds tends to detract from the enjoyment of the activity, and is completely unnecessary, anyway. So, if you're going to time yourself, do it once in a while, and don't let it get in the way of your enjoyment.

You may wish to start your programme with walks of, say, fifteen minutes duration. As you become fitter, you might want to build up gradually to thirty minutes or more. Once you can walk briskly for half an hour at a good, even, steady pace, then you may consider progressing to jogging.

Keep on running

If, for whatever reason, walking is the only form of exercise you take, that's fine. However, if you find you can progress to jogging without too much aggravation, then you're probably going to lose weight more efficiently in the long term. This is especially important where time is at a premium. If you've only got half an hour of exercise time at your disposal, then going just a little bit faster by breaking into a jog is very likely to reap rewards.

If you are new to jogging, then there are a few pointers that should help you get the most from your exercise sessions. First, don't go mad. What you should be looking to achieve is a good steady pace throughout the run. There is a tendency for individuals new to running to go off too fast, which may mean they need to stop prematurely. The trick is to start off at a pace that is actually lower than what you think you can sustain. If you still feel comfortable after five minutes, then you can step up the pace a little, but not before. As you get more experienced, you will be able to judge your natural pace much more easily and settle into this very quickly after a warm-up and stretch. Don't forget the warm-up and stretch!

When you begin to jog, you might find that you are unable to keep going for more than a few minutes at a time. That's fine. If you want, you can run for, say, three or four minutes, and then walk for a while. Start running again when you feel you are able to. Gradually, you should be able to build up the amount of time you are able to run without needing to stop, while gradually reducing the amount of recovery time you need in between. Whatever your ratio of jogging to walking, aim initially to be exercising for a total of about fifteen minutes. Again, you can gradually increase the total exercise time as you get fitter. Gradually you should build up to sessions lasting about half an hour.

Now, if you really get into the running thing, you might want to get a bit more adventurous. Maybe you could start jogging in a place that has some inclines. Take small steps and pump those arms up any incline, and hold yourself back a little on your way down – running down hill can be hard on the knees, back and ankles.

Another way to spice up your jog is to vary the pace. Perhaps you can experiment with picking up the pace for thirty seconds or so, going more slowly for a minute and then repeating this cycle. Maybe, if you are running in a place lined with lampposts or trees, you can use these as markers for your changes of pace. If you do find you have it in you to put little spurts in here and there, then the boost this is likely to give to fuel-burning can only do you good.

Aerobic – resistance training

Walking and jogging are what are known as 'aerobic' exercises. Basically, this means activities that are sustainable and demand the body to use a lot of oxygen. Other examples of aerobic activities include rowing, aerobics (surprise), cycling and step-machine exercise. Now, if you have any particular favourites in this bunch, then go for it. They make great substitutes for walking and jogging, their only downside is that they demand special equipment or access to a gym. If this isn't a barrier for you, then go ahead and do it.

At the other end of the spectrum to the aerobic exercises are the anaerobic exercises. These exercises do not demand much in the way of oxygen and include activities such as sprinting and weight training. At the beginning of this chapter we touched on the idea that strength training may have a significant role in weight loss. It's time to explain why.

Strength training – a new way to lose weight

Strength training is not traditionally regarded as an efficient way to lose weight. A strength training session may take 40 minutes or more, but the time spent exercising is much less. Maybe only a third or a quarter of the session time is spent actually exercising. Strength training is also hard work, it is a high intensity exercise and therefore will not burn much in the way of fat. It's no surprise then that strength training does not have a great reputation as a weight-loss aid. Also, for many women strength training often conjures up images of over-developed biceps and dwindling breasts. Many tend to shy away from strength training for this reason. However, despite the negative attitudes some of us have to strength training, there is good reason to believe it can be an effective tool in our effort to shed fat.

Muscle metabolism

Muscle is what is termed 'metabolically active'. Muscle burns calories all of the time, even when at rest. This means that the more muscle you have, the less likely you are to put on weight. The bad news is that, left to its own devices, muscle tissue tends to dwindle in time. Adults who do not maintain their muscle mass through strength training lose between 2.25–3 kg (5–7 lb) of muscle every ten years. Now, because muscles burn calories, this muscle loss leads to an inevitable drop in the body's metabolic rate. In fact, studies indicate that the metabolic rate drops by 2–5% every ten years, and loss of muscle tissue is probably the most important thing here. Now, this change may not sound like much, but it only takes very small changes in the metabolic rate to have a very profound effect on weight in the long term. For many individuals, maintaining muscle mass is key to lasting weight control.

The best way to keep the muscle bulk strong and healthy is strength training. It turns out that even relatively small changes in muscle mass can pay big dividends in the long term. Research has showed that just gaining just over 1 kg (3 lb) of muscle increases the metabolism by 7%. Individuals who gain muscle burn more calories, even when they're not active, and are less likely to accumulate fat as a result. To get this extra muscle doesn't necessarily take too much effort, either. One study showed that this sort of gain could be achieved by both men and women training for 25 minutes, three times a week for just eight weeks.

I know that the reality is you are unlikelty to want to take up a formalized, resistance-based regimes in order to lose weight, so Chris Williams and I have put together an exercise circuit for use in the home. This workout does contain strength-based exercises that are designed to help you at least maintain, and maybe even develop, your muscle mass, interspersed with aerobic exercises.

The home circuit

The home circuit is based on a series of exercises that alternate between resistance and aerobic-focused activities. If you complete the entire circuit three times, this should take about 20–30 minutes. If you can manage a couple of such sessions each week, then there's no doubt that you will be ensuring that you are going a long way towards serving your body's exercise needs.

Some technical points about the home circuit session

1. Perform the exercises in order, ensuring that you alternate between resistance and aerobic activities.

2. The exercises should be performed at a slow or moderate pace. Aim at a good consistent pace throughout, rather than getting through the session as quickly as possible.

3. Aim to do 10 repetitions of each of the resistance-based exercises, followed by 30 seconds of each aerobic exercise. The resistance exercises should be performed with a controlled, smooth action. If you are in the process of getting fit, you might want to restrict the aerobic exercise to something not too strenuous, such as actively marching on the spot.

4. Remember to keep breathing! During the resistance exercises it is common for individuals to restrict their breathing.

5. Don't forget to stretch before, and particularly after, the home circuit.

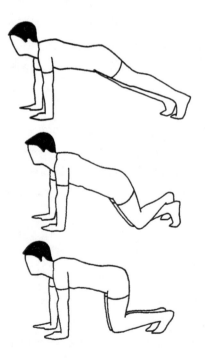

1. Press-ups

There's a choice of three here:

Full – keep your hips and knees straight. Your hands should be directly under your shoulders. Lower your body by bending your elbows until your chest is about 10 cm (4 in) from the floor. Push up again.

Half – similar to full press-ups, but the knees are on the ground set behind the hips.

Box – similar to the half, but the knees are directly under the hips.

2. Active march

March on the spot, lifting your knees high and pumping your arms.

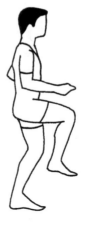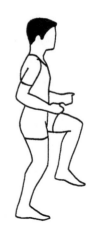

3. Sit-ups

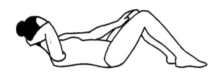

Lie with your back flat on the floor, with your knees bent and your feet flat. Place one hand on the thigh of the same side and the other hand behind your neck. Slowly lift your shoulder off the floor by squeezing your abdominal muscles. Curl your upper torso as you move forward towards your knees. Slide your hand along your thigh until your wrist gets to your knee. Hold briefly, and then lower yourself back to the ground slowly and in a controlled fashion. Keep your lower back in contact with the floor throughout this exercise, and do not pull your neck and head with the supporting hand.

4. Jog on the spot

Run on the spot, keeping both the upper and lower body relaxed.

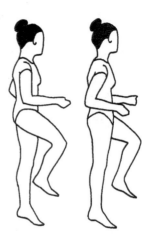

5. Bicep curls

Take two plastic 1½-litre (2½ pt) bottles of water, one in each hand. Hold the bottles with palms up and with your feet a shoulder-width apart and knees slightly bent. Bend your arms at the elbow, slowly raising your hands towards your chest. Pause briefly at the top and then lower the bottles with an easy, smooth action.

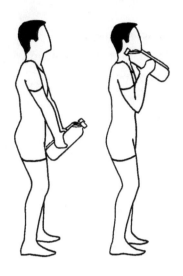

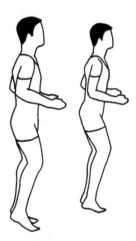

6 Ski jumps

Assume the ski position with feet slightly apart, knees slightly bent, your body slightly forward and your arms out in front. Jump slowly from side to side, cushioning your landing by bending your knees.

7. Squats

Starting with your feet a little more than a shoulder-width apart, toes pointed out at about 45 degrees and knees slightly bent. Sit down until your thighs are roughly parallel with the floor. Keep your knees over your ankles and swing your arms forward as you sit to keep your balance. Return to standing but do not lock your knees.

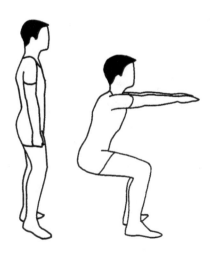

8. Spotty dog

Hold your hands above your head. From a standing start, kick your right leg forward and your left leg back as you bring your right arm forward and left arm up and back. Alternate this movement between the two sides.

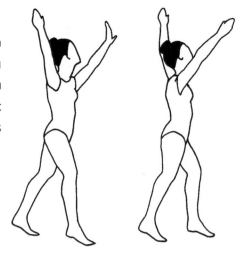

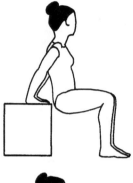

9. Dips

You will need a chair for this. Place the front of the chair behind you. Put your palms on the seat of the chair with your fingers pointing forward. Bend your knees and keep your feet flat on the floor. Take your weight on your arms and slowly bend your elbows to 90 degrees, lowering your hips towards the floor. Push back up again. Keep your back straight and close to the chair throughout.

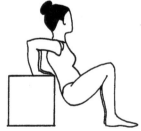

10. Jumping jacks

Stand with your feet a shoulder-width apart, your knees slightly bent and your hands at your side. Jump your legs out to the side as you simultaneously raise your arms out until your elbow is in line with your eyes. Jump back into the start position. You should not lock your knees during this exercise.

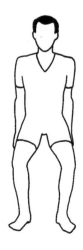

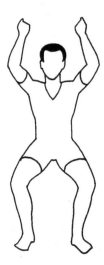

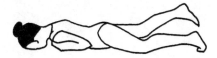

11. Back extensions

Lie face down on the floor and support your upper body by placing your hands palms-down under your chest. Bend your right leg slightly and lift it up off the floor, hold at the top for a count of one or two, and then lower. Repeat with your left leg. Keep the movements slow and rhythmical.

12. Jog on the spot

As with the jogging explained previously, but kick your heels up towards your buttocks.

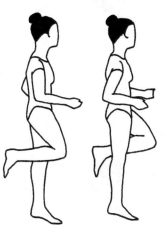

13. Lateral raises

Take two 1½-litre (2½ pt) plastic bottles of water, one in each hand. Stand with your feet a shoulder-width apart, with knees slightly bent. With arms straight, slowly raise them out to the sides until your elbow is in line with your eyes. Pause, and slowly return the bottles to your sides.

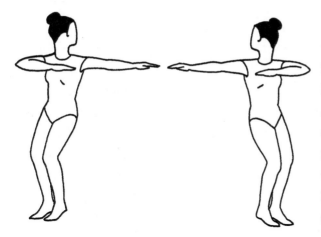

14. Twist jumps

Standing upright, with your knees slightly bent and your arms out in front, jump up and land your feet to the right and point your torso to the left. Use your arms to balance you. Repeat to the other side.

Case study

Angela P is a 35-year-old interior designer

Ever since I turned thirty I have been into exercise. I was a stone or so heavier than ideal, and controlling my weight was getting gradually more difficult. I felt I needed to do something. I joined the local gym and threw myself into a five-times-a-week exercise programme. I was not at all fit to begin with. I could not go fast but seemed to keep going for ages. Usually I would do thirty minutes on the treadmill, followed by ten minutes on the bike. I kept to the same routine for a month, and was disappointed to find that I only lost three pounds in this time. All that sweat for a measly three pounds!

One night I got chatting to a friend of my sister's who is a personal trainer. He explained to me where he thought I was going wrong, and roughed out another routine for me on the back of a napkin. He suggested that I only do 20 minutes-worth of aerobic exercise each day (either a run or cycle), but that I put more effort into it. He also advised my to start some light weights. I told him I didn't want to build up my muscles. He assured me I wouldn't. I really wanted something to shift, and was bored with my old regime, so decided to give it a go.

The next time I was in the gym, I asked one of the members of the gym staff to teach me a few weight-based exercises. He gave me a small pair of dumbbells and taught me exercises for my arms and shoulders. Then he showed me how to do proper press-ups and sit-ups. He put together a routine for me which literally only took 15 minutes but went through the whole body.

So, five times a week, I would do my new regime. Gradually, my running and cycling got stronger and faster, and so did my overall strength. As I got stronger, I started to lose weight. Eventually, I got down to my target weight in three or four months. I was thrilled, bearing in mind just how stuck my weight had been before.

Summary

- Although long periods of low intensity activity have been regarded as the best way to burn fat in the past, the latest evidence suggests that shorter periods of more strenuous activity and strength-based training are very useful tools for weight loss.

- For significant weight loss and health-related benefits, aim to take about 30 minutes worth of exercise, four times a week.

- Aim to be working at about 60-80% of your maximum heart rate (roughly equivalent to 220 – your age). If you can just snatch a conversation during exercise, then you are working hard enough, but not too hard.

- If you are new to exercise, walking is an ideal way to start your fitness campaign.

- If you are able, progress to jogging, as this is likely to help with both weight loss and health-related benefits.

- Resistance exercises can help weight loss by maintaining or developing muscle mass, which in turn impacts positively on the metabolism.

- A home exercise session based on both resistance and aerobic exercises offers a good convenient all-over workout.

Useful Information

Supplement Suppliers:

Advanced Herbals Ltd

Suppliers of hemp-seed oil by mail order.

Advanced Herbals Ltd
6 Forrest Street
Grangetown
Cardiff South Wales CF11 7EQ
Tel: 020 8938 3383

Rio Trading

Suppliers of stevia by mail order.

Rio Trading Ltd
2 Centenary Estate
Hughes Road
Brighton
East Sussex BN2 4AW
Tel: 01273 570987

VitaTech

Suppliers by mail order of the VitaTech range of supplements (including Hepranol, Thyranol, Glucoguard, Acidol and pepsin, Enzyme Forte, Replant, Acidophilus Forte, Permaguard and Canditrol.

VitaTech
Lakeside
180 Lifford Lane
Kings Norton
Birmingham B32 2HR
Tel: 0121 433 8729

Specialist Services:

Allergycare

Providers of allergy-related products, including specialist foods. Allergycare also has a countrywide food sensitivity testing service (electro-dermal testing) available through health food stores. Contact Allergycare for more details.

Allergycare Ltd
1 Church Square
Taunton
Somerset TA1 1SA
Tel: 01823 325022

BioLab

A specialist laboratory providing a range of tests, including the gut fermentation test and a test for stomach acidity. Tests need to be accessed via a practitioner. Contact BioLab for details.

BioLab
9 Weymouth Street
London W1N 3FF
Tel: 020 7636 5959

York Nutritional Laboratory

Providers of IgG blood testing for food sensitivity.

York Nutritional Laboratory
Murton Way
Osbalwick
York YO19 5US
Tel: 0800 0746184

Practitioner Bodies:

General Council and Register of Naturopaths

Provides a list of registered naturopathic practitioners.

General Council and Register of Naturopaths
Goswell House, 2 Goswell Road
Street, Somerset BA16 0JG
Tel: 01458 840072

MLD UK

MLD UK holds a register of practitioners qualified in manual lymphatic drainage therapy (MLD).

MLD UK, PO Box 149
Wallingford, Oxfordshire OX10 7LD

(Please send an SAE for a practitioner list)

Chris Williams can be contacted at Chris@williamshome.fsnet.co.uk or visit his web-site at
www.chriswilliams@health-hat.com

Dr John Briffa can be contacted at:

BodyWise
Woolaston House
25 Southwood Lane
Highgate
London N6 5ED

Or via e-mail at: woolaston.house@btinternet.com

Bibliography:

1. **Solved: The Riddle of Illness**,
   Stephen E Langer MD and James F Scheer:
   Keats Publishing 1984/1995

2. **Hypothyroidism: The Unsuspected Illness**, Broda Barnes MD and
   Lawrence Galton:
   Harper and Row 1976

3. **The Zone**, Barry Sears PhD with
   Bill Lawren: Regan Books 1995

4. **Dr Atkins' New Diet Revolution**,
   Robert C Atkins MD: Evans 1992/1999

5. **Potatoes not Prozac**,
   Kathleen DesMaisons PhD:
   Simon and Schuster 1998

6. **The Food Combining Diet**,
   Kathryn Marsden: Thorsons 1993

7. **Fats that Heal, Fats that Kill**,
   Dr Udo Erasmus: Alive Books 1987/1994

8. **Dr Braly's Food Allergy and Nutrition Revolution**, James Braly MD:
   Keats Publishing 1992

9. **The Complete Guide to Food Allergy and Intolerance**,
   Dr Jonathan Brostoff and Linda Gamlin:
   Bloomsbury 1989/1992

10. **Candida Albicans – A User's Guide to Treatment and Recovery**,
    Gill Jacobs: Optima 1990/1994

11. **The Practical Guide to Candida**,
    Jane McWhirter: All Hallows House
    Foundation 1995

12. **The Breath Book**,
    Stella Weller: Thorsons 1999

13. **Encyclopedia of Nutritional Supplements**,
    Michael Murray MD: Prima 1996

References

Chapter 1

(1) *Body image survey* Psychology Today 1997

(2) *Fat – Exploding the Myths* Lisa Colles: Carlton 1998

Chapter 2

(1) K D Brownwell, et al. *The effects of repeated cycles of weight loss and regain in rats.* Physiology and Behavior 1986; 38(4):459–464

(2) S N Steen, et al. *Metabolic effects of repeated cycles of weight loss and regain in adolescent wrestlers* Journal of the American Medical Association 1988; 26091:47–50

(3) USDA (United States Department of Agriculture): *Continuing survey of food intakes by individuals* (CSFII). Report #86-3, Hyattsville, MD, 1986.

(4) *'A square meal for Britain?'* Research by the Bateman Catering Organisation 1981

(5) Jenkins-David J A, et al. *Nibbling versus gorging: metabolic advantages of increased meal frequency.* New England Journal of Medicine 1989; 321(14): 929–934

Chapter 3

(1) Chalew S A, et al. *Diagnosis of reactive hypoglycaemia: pitfalls in the use of the oral glucose tolerance test* Southern Medical Journal 1986; 79: 285–287

(2) Kraft J. *Detection of diabetes mellitus in situ (occult diabetes)* Laboratory Medicine 1975 (Feb): 10

(3) Wurtman R J. *Neurochemical changes following high dose aspartame with dietary carbohydrates* New England Journal of Medicine 1983: 429–430

(4) Blundell J E, and Hill A J. *Paradoxical effects of an intense sweetener (aspartame) on appetite* The Lancet 1986; 1: 1092–1093

(5) Rogers P J, and Blundell J E. *Separating the actions of sweetness and calories: effects of saccharin and carbohydrates on hunger and food intake in human subjects* Physiology and Behaviour 1989; 45: 1093–1099

(6) Jorgensen H. *The influence of saccharin on blood sugar* Acta Physiologica Scandinavica 1950; 20: 33–37

(7) Anderson R A et al. *Effects of supplemental chromium on patients with symptoms of reactive hypoglycaemia* Metabolism 1987; 36(4): 351–355

(8) Anderson R A, et al. *Chromium supplementation in humans with hypoglycaemia* Federal Proceedings 1984; 43: 471

(9) Wimhurst J M and Manchester K L. *Comparison of the ability of magnesium and manganese to activate the key enzymes of glycolysis* FEBS Letters 1972; 27: 321–326

(10) Paolisso G, et al. *Daily magnesium supplements improve glucose handling in elderly subjects* American Journal of Clinical Nutrition 1992; 55: 1161–1167

Chapter 4

(1) *Hypothyroidism: The Unsuspected Illness* Broda Barnes MD and Lawrence Galton: Harper and Row 1976

(2) Olivieri O, et al. *Low selenium status in the elderly influences thyroid hormones* Clinical Science 1995; 89:637–642

(3) Behne D, et al. *1. Iodothyronine deiodinase activity after high selenium intake, relations between selenium and iodine metabolism in rats.* Journal of Nutrition 1992; 122:1542–1546

(4) Townsend Newsletter for Doctors, Dec 1989

Chapter 5

(1) *Fats that Heal, Fats that Kill* Dr Udo Erasmus: Alive Books, 1987/1994

(2) Atkinson R L et al. *The effects of conjugated linoleic acid in obese humans* (In preparation) (1998)

Chapter 6

(1) Randolph T G. *Masked food allergy as a factor in the development and persistence of obesity* Journal of Laboratory and Clinical Medicine 1947; 32: 1547

Chapter 7

(1) Chan R C Y, et al. *Competitive exclusion of uropathogens from human uroepitheilial cells by Lactobacillus whole cells and cell wall fragments* Infect. Immun. 1985; 47;84–89

(2) Poupard J A, et al. *Biology of the bifidobacteria* Bacteriological Reviews 1973; 136–165

(3) Shahani K M et al. *Natural antibiotic activity of lactobacillus acidophilus and bulgaricus II: Isolation of acidophilin from L. Acidophilus* Cult Dairy Prod J 1977; 12(2): 8–11

(4) Mann G V, et al. Spoerry A. *Studies of a surfactant and cholesteremia in the Masai* American Journal of Clinical Nutrition 1974; 464–469

(5) Plummer N. *The Lactic Acid Bacteria – Their Role in Human Health* BioMed Publications 1992

Chapter 8

(1) Faulstich J, et al. *Silibinin inhibition of amatoxin uptake in the perfused rat liver* Arzneim-Forsch Drug Research 1980; 30: 452–454

(2) Tuchweber B, et al. *Prevention by silibinin of phalloidin induced toxicity* Toxicol Appl Pharmacol 1979; 51: 265–275

(3) Feher J, Lang I, et al. *Free radicals in tissue damage in liver disease and therapeutic approach* Tokai J Exp Clin Med 1986; 11: 121–134 (4)

(4) Sonnenbichler J and Zetl I. *Stimulating influence of a flavonolignan derivative on proliferation, RNA synthesis and protein synthesis in liver cells.* Assessment and Management of Hepatobiliary Disease Berlin: Springer-Verlag 1987

Index